ATRIAL AND VENTRICULAR SEPTAL DEFECTS

MOLECULAR DETERMINANTS, IMPACT OF ENVIRONMENTAL FACTORS AND NON-SURGICAL INTERVENTIONS

CARDIOLOGY RESEARCH AND CLINICAL DEVELOPMENTS

Additional books in this series can be found on Nova's website under the Series tab.

Additional E-books in this series can be found on Nova's website under the E-book tab.

CARDIOLOGY RESEARCH AND CLINICAL DEVELOPMENTS

ATRIAL AND VENTRICULAR SEPTAL DEFECTS

MOLECULAR DETERMINANTS, IMPACT OF ENVIRONMENTAL FACTORS AND NON-SURGICAL INTERVENTIONS

STEVEN A. LARKIN
EDITOR

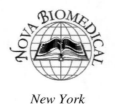

New York

For permission to use material from this book please contact us:
Telephone 631-231-7269; Fax 631-231-8175
Web Site: http://www.novapublishers.com

NOTICE TO THE READER

The Publisher has taken reasonable care in the preparation of this book, but makes no expressed or implied warranty of any kind and assumes no responsibility for any errors or omissions. No liability is assumed for incidental or consequential damages in connection with or arising out of information contained in this book. The Publisher shall not be liable for any special, consequential, or exemplary damages resulting, in whole or in part, from the readers' use of, or reliance upon, this material. Any parts of this book based on government reports are so indicated and copyright is claimed for those parts to the extent applicable to compilations of such works.

Independent verification should be sought for any data, advice or recommendations contained in this book. In addition, no responsibility is assumed by the publisher for any injury and/or damage to persons or property arising from any methods, products, instructions, ideas or otherwise contained in this publication.

This publication is designed to provide accurate and authoritative information with regard to the subject matter covered herein. It is sold with the clear understanding that the Publisher is not engaged in rendering legal or any other professional services. If legal or any other expert assistance is required, the services of a competent person should be sought. FROM A DECLARATION OF PARTICIPANTS JOINTLY ADOPTED BY A COMMITTEE OF THE AMERICAN BAR ASSOCIATION AND A COMMITTEE OF PUBLISHERS.

Additional color graphics may be available in the e-book version of this book.

Library of Congress Cataloging-in-Publication Data

ISBN: 978-1-62618-326-1

Library of Congress Control Number: 2013933805

Published by Nova Science Publishers, Inc. † New York

CONTENTS

PREFACE

In this book, the authors have gathered and present topical research in the study of the molecular determinants, impact of environmental factors and non-surgical interventions relating to atrial and ventricular septal defects. Topics discussed in this compilation include the molecular mechanisms of ventricular septal defects; maternal characteristics and use of drugs and septum heart defects in children; non-surgical closure of atrial septal defects in children; and the etiology and percutaneous closure of atrial and ventricular septal defects.

Chapter 1 - Ventricular septal defect is the most common type of congenital heart disease. Despite of the many advances in the authors' understanding of cardiac development and many genes related to cardiac development identified, the fundamental etiology for the majority of cases of congenital heart disease remains unknown. Ventricular septal defect is a multifactorial complex disease, with environmental and genetic factors playing important roles. A number of causative genes of ventricular septal defect have been found. The molecular mechanisms of ventricular septal defect may include mutations in components of the cardiac gene network, altered haemodynamics, regulatory pathway of cardiac genes, microRNA dysfunction, epignetics, adult congenital heart diseases and so on. Conclusions: The molecular basis of ventricular septal defect is an exciting and rapidly evolving field. The continuing advances in the understanding of the molecular mechanisms of ventricular septal defect will hopefully result in improved genetic counseling and care of affected individuals and their families. This review summarizes normal cardiac development, and outlines the recent discoveries of the genetic causes of ventricular septal defect, and provides possible strategies for exploring them.

Chapter 2 - Congenital cardiac septum defects are common malformations. A large number of possible causal factors have been published, mainly from retrospective case-control studies. The present analysis is based on Swedish health registers and investigates some maternal risk factors for ventricular (VSD) and atrial (ASD) septum defects. A total of 7308 children with septum defects were identified with the use of three different national registers and risk factors were ascertained from the Medical Birth Register and consist of data collected in early pregnancy.

Maternal age and parity have weak effects on the risk for septum defects, similar for VSD and ASD. Maternal smoking in early pregnancy was associated with an increased risk for ASD but a slightly decreased risk for VSD. Maternal overweight or obesity was associated with an increased risk for ASD but not for VSD. Couple subfertility (evaluated from number of years of unwanted childlessness) was a stronger risk factor for ASD than for VSD. Maternal pre-existing diabetes (mainly type 1) was a strong factor with a three times increased risk for any septum defect, highest for combined VSD+ASD, intermediate for only ASD, and lowest for only VSD.

Children with a septum defect were born preterm more often than other children and the highest odds ratio for preterm birth was seen for ASD. There was an excess of females, most pronounced for combined VSD+ASD. There was an excess of multiple births, notably for ASD.

Maternal use of a wide spectrum of drugs was analyzed with adjustments made for year of birth, maternal age, parity, smoking, and BMI. Increased risks were seen for a number of drug categories. Use of aminosalicylic acid drugs was associated with an increased risk (OR = 1.76) and also use of immunosuppressive drugs (OR = 3.31), both may at least partly be due to underlying pathology. This is probably the case also for the increased risk after use of thyroxin (OR = 1.22). An increased risk was also seen after antihypertensive drugs (OR = 1.61), anticonvulsants (OR = 1.74), tricyclic antidepressants (OR = 1.95) and paroxetine (OR = 2.15). No effect was seen for other antidepressants or from NSAIDs (including ibuprofen). An increased risk after use of vitamin B12 could be explained by concomitant drug use.

To conclude, some maternal characteristics and chronic diseases were risk factors for cardiac septum defects in the child and the maternal use of a few drugs may also carry a risk.

Chapter 3 - There are four types of *atrial septal* defects (ASDs) namely, ostium secundum, ostium primum, sinus venosus and coronary sinus ASDs. Patent foramen ovale (PFO) is present in nearly one third of normal population, thus making the PFO a normal variant, although it may become important in certain situations and will not be the subject of this review. In this review management of only ostium secundum ASDs is discussed. Whereas surgical intervention was used in the past, transcatheter methods are currently used for closure of ostium secundum ASDs. A large number of devices have been developed over the last three and one-half decades. Some of the devices have been discontinued and others modified and redesigned. Clinical trials have been undertaken with a large number of devices and feasibility, safety and effectiveness of these devices in occluding the ASD have been demonstrated. At the present time however, Amplatzer Septal Occluder, Amplatzer Cribriform Device and HELEX devices are the only devices that are approved for general clinical use by the FDA. The experience with Amplatzer for most defects has been encouraging. HELEX device is only useful in small to medium-sized defects. Historical aspects of device development, indications for intervention, the method of device implantation, immediate and follow-up results (along with complications), including the authors' personal experience with Amplatzer device in over 150 patients and a comparison with surgery will be presented. It may be concluded that Amplatzer device may be the best available option at the present time. Careful attention to the details of the technique is mandatory to achieve a successful outcome.

Chapter 4 - Atrial and ventricular septal defects (AVSD) are the most frequent congenital heart defects, affecting a 0.5% of new-borns. Their etiology includes a variety of causes, from genetic or genomic variation to the exposure to environment factors.

Among AVSD there are two well differentiated scenarios: 1) syndromic AVSD (Down syndrome or Holt-Oram syndrome) where genetic disturbances are the main reason for the development of the condition, and 2) non syndromic AVSD where the interaction between genetic predisposition and environment factors affects critically biological systems during heart development.

Genetic predisposition is not always fully characterized although some specific genetic features like carrying MDR1 3435CT/TT genotype or NNMT A allele have been proven an additional risk for developing non syndromic AVSD. This risk can be higher when some types of environment factors get combined, including cigarette smoking, benzodyacepines, alcohol and serotonin reuptake inhibitors consumption and the exposure to air pollution. All of these are present often in daily life, constituting a reason for great concern.

The association between environment factors and the development of AVSD has been repeteadly shown in different studies; for instance, cigarette smoking during pregnancy causes a three-fold increase in the risk of AVSD. The majority of thes studies are, however, retrospective epidemiological studies, what carries a great limitation for the interpretation of results. Therefore, prospective cohort studies would be paramount to get more definite conclusions about the influence of environment factors in the development of AVSD.

The extraordinary development of medical devices has made possible the percutaneous (non surgical) treatment of atrial and ventricular septal defects in many cases.

In the case of atrial septal defects (ASD), percutaneous closure is mainly indicated for ostium secundum defects although other types of ASD can also be treated percutaneously. In order to establish correctly the indication of closure both right cardiac catheterization and echocardiography are critical, not only for patient selection but for guidance and assistance during the closure procedure.

Several ASD ocluders are clinically available (Amplatzer[tm], Gore Helex[tm], STARFlex[tm], Premere[tm]...) all of them consisting of two discs separated by a waist. In general, the vast majority of ASD can be treated percutaneously with reasonably small sheats (12 french or less). Success rates are very high (98-99% after three months of follow up) and complications (device embolization, pericardial effusion or trombosis) are usually below 1%.

Regarding ventricular septal defects (VSD) percutaneous treatment is not so widely used. Post-myocardial infarction VSD with a very high surgical risk and selected cases of perimembranous VSD are the ones treated more commonly. With a correct case selection, percutaneous closure of VSD is a safe and feasible procedure, although small residual left to right shunts are observed in a relatively high percentage of patients.

In: Atrial and Ventricular Septal Defects   ISBN: 978-1-62618-326-1
Editor: Steven A. Larkin   © 2013 Nova Science Publishers, Inc.

Chapter 1

MOLECULAR MECHANISMS OF VENTRICULAR SEPTAL DEFECT

Jing-bin Huang, Jian Liang[*]*, Xin Deng, Wen-sen Wu and Xiao-fang Zhao*

Department of Cardiothoracic Surgery,
Ruikang Hospital Affiliated to Guangxi University of Chinese Medicine,
Nanning, Guangxi Zhuang Autonomous Region, China

ABSTRACT

Ventricular septal defect is the most common type of congenital heart disease. Despite of the many advances in our understanding of cardiac development and many genes related to cardiac development identified, the fundamental etiology for the majority of cases of congenital heart disease remains unknown. Ventricular septal defect is a multifactorial complex disease, with environmental and genetic factors playing important roles. A number of causative genes of ventricular septal defect have been found. The molecular mechanisms of ventricular septal defect may include mutations in components of the cardiac gene network, altered haemodynamics, regulatory pathway of cardiac genes, microRNA dysfunction, epignetics, adult congenital heart diseases and so on. Conclusions: The molecular basis of ventricular septal defect is an exciting and rapidly evolving field. The continuing advances in the understanding of the molecular mechanisms of ventricular septal defect

[*] Corresponding author: Jian Liang MD, E-mail:hjb010222@163.com.

will hopefully result in improved genetic counseling and care of affected individuals and their families. This review summarizes normal cardiac development, and outlines the recent discoveries of the genetic causes of ventricular septal defect, and provides possible strategies for exploring them.

Keywords: Congenital heart disease, ventricular septal defect, molecular mechanism; genetics

INTRODUCTION

Congenital heart disease (CHD) is the most common type of birth defect, affecting 1% of all live births, and is the leading non-infectious cause of death in the first year of life [1, 2]. Ventricular septal defect is the most common type of congenital heart disease. Despite of the many advances in our understanding of cardiac development and many genes related to cardiac development identified, the fundamental etiology for the majority of cases of congenital heart disease remains unknown. CHD is a multifactorial complex disease, with environmental and genetic factors playing important roles. It has been recognized that environmental factors insults during fetal development increase the risk of CHD, including viral infections with rubella [3], exposure to chemical teratogens such as retinoic acid, lithium, dilantin [4] and halogenated hydrocarbon [5] and maternal diseases including diabetes and systemic lupus erythematosus [1, 6]. Epidemiologic studies of CHD have demonstrated an increased recurrence risk for cardiac malformations in sequent pregnancies, supporting the existence of gene predispositions.

Great progress in molecular genetics and developmental biology has been made. Current genetic techniques for evaluation of congenital heart defects include cytogenetic techniques, fluorescence *in situ* hybridization (FISH), DNA mutation analysis. Most methods employ polymerase chain reaction–based assays. Indirect screening methods, such as denaturing high-performance liquid chromatography or single-strand conformation polymorphism have been used extensively. More expensive exon-by-exon sequencing of genomic DNA has recently emerged [7, 8]. It has been accepted that the intricate process of cardiac morphogenesis is controlled by a network of highly conserved genetic and molecular pathways. The origins of CHD are diverse, such as abnormal chromosome structure (e.g. duplication or deletion), gene mutations, single nucleotide polymorphisms, abnormal RNA, epigenetics and so on, and they are summarized as Figure 1.

In humans, heart development begins at 15 to 16 days of gestation with the migration of precardiac stem cells, in five steps:(1) migration of precardiac cells from the primitive streak and assembly of the paired cardiac crescents at the myocardial plate, (2) coalescence of the cardiac crescents to form the primitive heart tube, establishment of the definitive heart, (3) cardiac looping, assurance of proper alignment of the future cardiac chambers, (4) septation and heart chambers formation, and (5) development of the cardiac conduction system and coronary vasculature [9-11]. The establishment of left-right asymmetry is very important to the normal development of heart [12, 13]. Secreted FGF, BMP, Nodal, and Wnt act as input signal of symmetric cardiac morphogenesis, BMP2, FGF8, Shh/Ihh and Nodal function as positive regulators, whereas Wnt and Ser are negative regulators [14-16]. The cardiogenic plate-specific expressed genes NKX2. 5SRF, GATA4, TBX5 and HAND2 compose the core regulatory network of cardiac morphogenesis, controlling heart looping, left-right symmetry and chambers formation. SRF regulates the differentiation of coronary vascular smooth muscle cells [17, 18]. Genes that involved in epicardial development include FOG-2, vascular cell adhesion molecule 1, integrins, erythropoietin, and erythropoietin receptor. Specific genes such as the NOTCH receptor, Jagged (JAG), WNT, transforming growth factor beta 2 (TGF ß2) and bone morphogenic proteins have been implicated in cardiac neural crest development in the mouse [12, 19-21]. Retinoic acid signal pathway is involved in the regulation of cardiac looping. Complex signal pathways are implicated in the crosstalk between endocardium and myocardium to form endocardial cushion and heart valves, including VEGF, NFATc1, Notch, Wnt/ß-catenin, BMP/TGF-ß, EGF, erbB NF1 signal pathways [10, 22-24].

MOLECULAR MECHANISMS OF VENTRICULAR SEPTAL DEFECT

Causative Genes of Ventricular Septal Defect

The etiological factors of many genetic syndromes and familial CHD have been identified, but the genetic basis of majority of "sporadic" CHD remains unknown. With the progress in molecular genetics and developmental biology, many genes associated heart development have been identified. When searching computer databases such as NCBI Gene Bank for "heart or cardiac", we can indentify 1970 loci in human. Search for "(heart or cardiac) and development", limited to human, 1241 genes were found. A number of selected congenital heart defects and genetic syndromes have been found to be associated with mutations in a variety of single genes. The mutations were found only in affected individuals, were not present in control samples, and were demonstrated to change protein structure or function. Disease genes of ventricular septal defect identified to date are summarized in Table 1, and the functions of these causative genes are summarized as following [25].

Table 1. Causative genes of VSD

Causative genes	Official full name	Gene type	Chromosome location
GATA4	GATA binding protein 4	Protein coding	8p23.1-p22
NKX2-5	NK2 homeobox 5	Protein coding	5q34
VEGFA	Vascular endothelial growth factor A	Protein coding	6p12
CITED2	Cbp/p300-interacting transactivator, with Glu/Asp-rich carboxy-terminal domain, 2	Protein coding	6q23.3
PSEN1	Presenilin 1	Protein coding	14q24.3
NOTCH1	Notch 1	Protein coding	9q34.3
CACNA1C	Calcium channel, voltage-dependent, L type, alpha 1C subunit	Protein coding	12p13.3
NFATC1	Nuclear factor of activated T-cells, cytoplasmic, calcineurin-dependent 1	Protein coding	18q23
RTN4	Reticulon 4	Protein coding	2p16.3
GATA6	GATA binding protein 6	Protein coding	18q11.1-q11.2
TBX5	T-Box 5	Protein coding	12q24.1
SALL4	Sal-like 4	Protein coding	20q13.2
TBX1	T-Box 1	Protein coding	22q11.21

Causative genes	Official full name	Gene type	Chromosome location
MKKS	McKusick-Kaufman syndrome	Protein coding	20p12
DGCR8	DiGeorge syndrome critical region gene 8	Protein coding	22q11.2
DGCR2	DiGeorge syndrome critical region gene 2	Protein coding	22q11.21
DGCR14	DiGeorge syndrome critical region gene 14	Protein coding	22q11.2
DGCR6	DiGeorge syndrome critical region gene 6	Protein coding	22q11
IRX4	Iroquois homeobox 4	Protein coding	5p15.3
DGCR	DiGeorge syndrome chromosome region	Other	22q11.21-q11.23

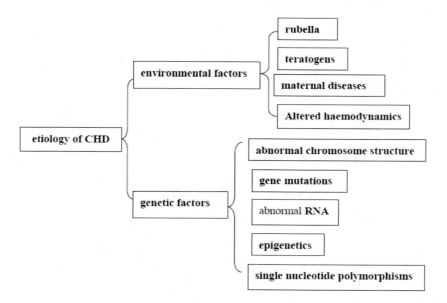

Figure 1. Eteology of CHD.

For example, NKX2-5, Homeobox-containing genes play critical roles in regulating tissue-specific gene expression essential for tissue differentiation, as well as determining the temporal and spatial patterns of development. It has been demonstrated that a Drosophila homeobox-containing gene called 'tinman' is expressed in the developing dorsal vessel and in the equivalent of the vertebrate heart. Mutations in tinman result in loss of heart formation in the embryo, suggesting that tinman is essential for Drosophila heart formation. Furthermore, abundant expression of Csx, the presumptive mouse homolog of tinman, is observed only in the heart from the time of cardiac differentiation. CSX, the human homolog of murine Csx, has a homeodomain sequence identical to that of Csx and is expressed only in the heart, again suggesting that CSX plays an important role in human heart formation. Studies have recently shown that nonsyndromic CHD can result from single-gene defects. Schott et al identified mutations in *NKX2.5* in 4 kindreds with atrial septal defects and atrioventricular conduction delay without other apparent syndromic features. The mutations were found only in affected individuals, were not present in control samples, and were demonstrated to change protein structure or function [26-28].

Noonan Syndrome is a genetic multiple malformation disorder that includes short stature, typical facial dysmorphism, webbed neck, chest deformity, and cardiovascular abnormalities. The cardiac involvement is observed in 80% to 90% of affected individuals, with valvar pulmonic stenosis and hypertrophic cardiomyopathy being the most common. Other congenital heart defects observed in Noonan Syndrome are secundum atrial septal defect, atrioventricular septal defect, mitral valve abnormalities, aortic coarctation, and tetralogy of Fallot. Noonan Syndrome is genetically heterogeneous, which means that there are at least 3 Noonan Syndrome disease genes, *PTPN11*, *SOS1*, and *KRAS* [29]. It is *PTPN11*, which encodes a protein tyrosine phosphatase called SHP-2. SHP-2 plays an important role in signal transduction for a wide variety of biological processes, including the formation of the semilunar valves. Mutations in the *PTPN11* gene are observed in 40% to 50% of Noonan Syndrome patients [25, 30].

Functions of the Causative Genes of Ventricular Septal Defect

The causative genes of ventricular septal defect are described as follows:

GATA4, Official Full Name: GATA Binding Protein 4

This gene encodes a member of the GATA family of zinc-finger transcription factors. Members of this family recognize the GATA motif which is present in the promoters of many genes. This protein is thought to regulate genes involved in embryogenesis and in myocardial differentiation and function. Mutations in this gene have been associated with cardiac septal defects [31-35].

NKX2-5, Official Full NameNK2 Homeobox 5

This gene encodes a homeobox-containing transcription factor. This transcription factor functions in heart formation and development. Mutations in this gene cause atrial septal defect with atrioventricular conduction defect, and also tetralogy of Fallot, which are both heart malformation diseases. Mutations in this gene can also cause congenital hypothyroidism non-goitrous type 5, a non-autoimmune condition. Alternative splicing results in multiple transcript variants [36-39].

VEGFA, Official Full Name: Vascular Endothelial Growth Factor

This gene is a member of the PDGF/VEGF growth factor family and encodes a protein that is often found as a disulfide linked homodimer. This protein is a glycosylated mitogen that specifically acts on endothelial cells and has various effects, including mediating increased vascular permeability, inducing angiogenesis, vasculogenesis and endothelial cell growth, promoting cell migration, and inhibiting apoptosis. Elevated levels of this protein is linked to POEMS syndrome, also known as Crow-Fukase syndrome. Mutations in this gene have been associated with proliferative and nonproliferative diabetic retinopathy. Alternatively spliced transcript variants, encoding either freely secreted or cell-associated isoforms, have been characterized. There is also evidence for the use of non-AUG (CUG) translation initiation sites upstream of, and in-frame with the first AUG, leading to additional isoforms [40-44].

CITED2, Official Full Name: Cbp/p300-Interacting Transactivator, with Glu/Asp-rich Carboxy-terminal Domain, 2

The protein encoded by this gene inhibits transactivation of HIF1A-induced genes by competing with binding of hypoxia-inducible factor 1-alpha to p300-CH1. Mutations in this gene are a cause of cardiac septal defects. Alternatively spliced transcript variants encoding multiple isoforms have been observed for this gene [45-48].

PSEN1, Official Full Name: Presenilin 1

Alzheimer's disease (AD) patients with an inherited form of the disease carry mutations in the presenilin proteins (PSEN1; PSEN2) or in the amyloid precursor protein (APP). These disease-linked mutations result in increased production of the longer form of amyloid-beta (main component of amyloid deposits found in AD brains). Presenilins are postulated to regulate APP processing through their effects on gamma-secretase, an enzyme that cleaves APP. Also, it is thought that the presenilins are involved in the cleavage of the Notch receptor, such that they either directly regulate gamma-secretase activity or themselves are protease enzymes. Several alternatively spliced transcript variants encoding different isoforms have been identified for this gene, the full-length nature of only some have been determined [49-52].

NOTCH1, Official Full Name: Notch 1

This gene encodes a member of the Notch family. Members of this Type 1 transmembrane protein family share structural characteristics including an extracellular domain consisting of multiple epidermal growth factor-like (EGF) repeats, and an intracellular domain consisting of multiple, different domain types. Notch family members play a role in a variety of developmental processes by controlling cell fate decisions. The Notch signaling network is an evolutionarily conserved intercellular signaling pathway which regulates interactions between physically adjacent cells. In Drosophilia, notch interaction with its cell-bound ligands (delta, serrate) establishes an intercellular signaling pathway that plays a key role in development. Homologues of the notch-ligands have also been identified in human, but precise interactions between these ligands and the human notch homologues remain to be determined. This protein is cleaved in the trans-Golgi network, and presented on the cell surface as a heterodimer. This protein functions as a receptor for membrane bound ligands, and may play multiple roles during development [53-57].

CACNA1C, Official Full Name: Calcium Channel, Voltage-dependent, L Type, Alpha 1C Subunit

This gene encodes an alpha-1 subunit of a voltage-dependent calcium channel. Calcium channels mediate the influx of calcium ions into the cell upon membrane polarization. The alpha-1 subunit consists of 24 transmembrane segments and forms the pore through which ions pass into the cell. The calcium channel consists of a complex of alpha-1, alpha-2/delta, beta, and gamma subunits in a 1:1:1:1 ratio. There are multiple isoforms of each of these proteins, either encoded by different genes or the result of alternative splicing of transcripts. The protein encoded by this gene binds to and is inhibited by dihydropyridine. Alternative splicing results in many transcript variants encoding different proteins. Some of the predicted proteins may not produce functional ion channel subunits [58-62].

NFATC1, Official Full Name: Nuclear Factor of Activated T-Cells, Cytoplasmic, Calcineurin-dependent 1

The product of this gene is a component of the nuclear factor of activated T cells DNA-binding transcription complex. This complex consists of at least two components: a preexisting cytosolic component that translocates to the nucleus upon T cell receptor (TCR) stimulation, and an inducible nuclear component. Proteins belonging to this family of transcription factors play a central role in inducible gene transcription during immune response. The product of this gene is an inducible nuclear component. It functions as a major molecular target for the immunosuppressive drugs such as cyclosporin A. Five transcript variants encoding distinct isoforms have been identified for this gene. Different isoforms of this protein may regulate inducible expression of different cytokine genes [63-68].

RTN4, Official Full Name: Reticulon 4

This gene belongs to the family of reticulon encoding genes. Reticulons are associated with the endoplasmic reticulum, and are involved in neuroendocrine secretion or in membrane trafficking in neuroendocrine cells. The product of this gene is a potent neurite outgrowth inhibitor which may also help block the regeneration of the central nervous system in higher vertebrates. Alternatively spliced transcript variants derived both from differential splicing and differential promoter usage and encoding different isoforms have been identified [69-73].

GATA6, Official Full Name: GATA Binding Protein 6

This gene is a member of a small family of zinc finger transcription factors that play an important role in the regulation of cellular differentiation and organogenesis during vertebrate development. This gene is expressed during early embryogenesis and localizes to endo- and mesodermally derived cells during later embryogenesis and thereby plays an important role in gut, lung, and heart development. Mutations in this gene are associated with several congenital defects [74-77].

TBX5, Official Full Name: T-Box 5

This gene is a member of a phylogenetically conserved family of genes that share a common DNA-binding domain, the T-box. T-box genes encode transcription factors involved in the regulation of developmental processes. This gene is closely linked to related family member T-box 3 (ulnar mammary syndrome) on human chromosome 12. The encoded protein may play a role in heart development and specification of limb identity. Mutations in this gene have been associated with Holt-Oram syndrome, a developmental disorder affecting the heart and upper limbs. Several transcript variants encoding different isoforms have been described for this gene [78-81].

SALL4, Official Full Name: Sal-like 4

The protein encoded by this gene may be a zinc finger transcription factor. Defects in this gene are a cause of Duane-radial ray syndrome (DRRS) [82-86].

TBX1, Official Full Name: T-Box 1

This gene is a member of a phylogenetically conserved family of genes that share a common DNA-binding domain, the T-box. T-box genes encode transcription factors involved in the regulation of developmental processes. This gene product shares 98% amino acid sequence identity with the mouse ortholog. DiGeorge syndrome (DGS) /velocardiofacial syndrome (VCFS), a common congenital disorder characterized by neural-crest-related developmental defects, has been associated with deletions of chromosome 22q11.2, where this gene has been mapped. Studies using mouse models of DiGeorge syndrome suggest a major role for this gene in the molecular etiology of DGS/VCFS. Several alternatively spliced transcript variants encoding different isoforms have been described for this gene [87-91].

MKKS, Official Full Name: McKusick-Kaufman Syndrome

This gene encodes a protein which shares sequence similarity with other members of the chaperonin family. The encoded protein may have a role in protein folding, processing and assembly. Mutations in this gene have been observed in patients with Bardet-Biedl syndrome type 6 and McKusick-Kaufman syndrome. Alternative splicing results in multiple transcript variants [92-96].

DGCR8, Official Full Name: DiGeorge Syndrome Critical Region Gene 8

This gene encodes a subunit of the microprocessor complex which mediates the biogenesis of microRNAs from the primary microRNA transcript. The encoded protein is a double-stranded RNA binding protein that functions as the non-catalytic subunit of the microprocessor complex. This

protein is required for binding the double-stranded RNA substrate and facilitates cleavage of the RNA by the ribonuclease III protein, Drosha. Alternate splicing results in multiple transcript variants [97-101].

DGCR2, Official Full Name: DiGeorge Syndrome Critical Region Gene 2

Deletions of the 22q11.2 have been associated with a wide range of developmental defects (notably DiGeorge syndrome, velocardiofacial syndrome, conotruncal anomaly face syndrome and isolated conotruncal cardiac defects) classified under the acronym CATCH 22. The DGCR2 gene encodes a novel putative adhesion receptor protein, which could play a role in neural crest cells migration, a process which has been proposed to be altered in DiGeorge syndrome. Alternative splicing results in multiple transcript variants [102-104].

DGCR14, Official Full Name: DiGeorge Syndrome Critical Region Gene 14

This gene is located within the minimal DGS critical region (MDGCR) thought to contain the gene(s) responsible for a group of developmental disorders. These disorders include DiGeorge syndrome, velocardiofacial syndrome, conotruncal anomaly face syndrome, and some familial or sporadic conotruncal cardiac defects which have been associated with microdeletion of 22q11.2. The encoded protein may be a component of C complex spliceosomes, and the orthologous protein in the mouse localizes to the nucleus [105-108].

DGCR6, Official Full Name: DiGeorge Syndrome Critical Region Gene 6

DiGeorge syndrome, and more widely, the CATCH 22 syndrome, are associated with microdeletions in chromosomal region 22q11.2. The product of this gene shares homology with the Drosophila melanogaster gonadal protein, which participates in gonadal and germ cell development, and with the gamma-1 subunit of human laminin. This gene is a candidate for involvement in DiGeorge syndrome pathology and in schizophrenia [109-112].

IRX4, Official Full Name: Iroquois Homeobox 4

IRX4 is expressed specifically in the prostate and heart. IRX4 was the first identified cardiac transcription factor that is restricted to the ventricles at all stages of heart development. Irx4-deficient mice show ventricular dysfunction and develop cardiomyopathy. IRX4 had a potential causative impact on the development of congenital heart disease, particularly ventricular septal defect [113-117].

DGCR, Official Full Name: DiGeorge Syndrome Chromosome Region

DiGeorge syndrome (DGS) comprises hypocalcemia arising from parathyroid hypoplasia, thymic hypoplasia, and outflow tract defects of the heart. Disturbance of cervical neural crest migration into the derivatives of the pharyngeal arches and pouches can account for the phenotype. Most cases result from a deletion of chromosome 22q11.2 (the DiGeorge syndrome chromosome region, or DGCR). Several genes are lost including the putative transcription factor TUPLE1 which is expressed in the appropriate distribution. This deletion may present with a variety of phenotypes: Shprintzen, or velocardiofacial, syndrome (VCFS; MIM 192430); conotruncal anomaly face (or Takao syndrome); and isolated outflow tract defects of the heart including tetralogy of Fallot, truncus arteriosus, and interrupted aortic arch. A collective acronym CATCH22 has been proposed for these differing presentations. A small number of cases of DGS have defects in other chromosomes, notably 10p13 (see MIM 601362). In the mouse, a transgenic Hox A3 (Hox 1.5) knockout produces a phenotype similar to DGS as do the teratogens retinoic acid and alcohol [118-120].

PATHOGENIC MECHANISMS OF VENTRICULAR SEPTAL DEFECT

Phenotypes of CHD vary from small ASD and VSD, which may go undetected throughout life, to large ASD and VSD, which are significantly symptomatic. Clinically significant anomalies range from persistence of fetal circulation (e.g., patent ductus arteriosus) to complex defects such as transposition of the great vessels, single ventricle anomaly, hypoplastic left heart syndrome, and complex variants of heterotaxy. The etiological factors of many genetic syndromes and familial CHD have been identified, but the genetic basis of majority of "sporadic" CHD remains unknown. It is hypothesized that susceptibility resulted from single nucleotide polymorphisms or key gene(s), with the interaction of environmental factors, which disturb normal cardiac development, result in cardiac defects. There are six causative mechanisms according to pathogenetic classification of congenital cardiovascular malformations: ectomesenchymal tissue migration abnormalities (causing conotruncal malformations and aortic arch anomalies); intracardiac blood flow defects (causing septal defects and left or right heart obstructive malformations); cell death abnormalities (causing septal defects and valve abnormalities); extra cellular matrix abnormalities (causing atrioventricular canal defects); abnormal targeted growth (causing partial or total anomalous pulmonary venous return and cor triatriatum); and abnormal situs and looping (causing left–right positioning problems) [121, 122].

Mutations in Components of the Cardiac Gene Network Cause Ventricular Septal Defect

Heart development is controlled by a highly conserved network of transcription factors that connect signaling pathways with genes of muscle growth, patterning, and contractility. The core transcription factor network consists of *NKX2, MEF2, GATA, TBX,* and *Hand.* Dozens of other transcription factors contribute to cardiogenesis, in many cases by serving as accessory factors for these core regulators. Autoregulatory and cross regulatory of the cardiac gene network maintain the cardiac phenotype once the network has been activated by upstream inductive signals. Mutations in components of the cardiac gene Network cause ventricular septal defect [123,124].

Mutations in *NKX2.5* cause a spectrum of congenital heart defects, including atrial-septal defects (ASDs), ventricular-septal defects (VSDs), and cardiac conduction abnormalities. Mutations in TBX5 cause the congenital disease Holt–Oram syndrome, which is characterized by truncations of the upper limbs and heart malformations [125, 126]. Mutations in *GATA4*, some of which disrupt its interaction with *TBX5*, cause ASDs and VSDs. In mouse models, haploinsufficiency for Nkx2-5 or Tbx5 resulted in an increased incidence of structural heart disease, confirming that normal heart development is sensitive to small changes in expression levels of Nkx2-5 and Tbx5. GATA4 also is an essential, dosage-dependent regulator of cardiac morphogenesis. The missense mutation in Gata4 specifically disrupted the Gata4-Tbx5 interaction while maintaining its ability to interact with Nkx2.5. In previous studies, Tbx5 had been shown to interact with Nkx2.5, demonstrating that all three transcription factors could physically interact *in vitro*. In summary, a mutation in any of these three genes can result in human

CSD and suggests that these three genes may work to direct common molecular pathways critical for cardiac septum formation. [127, 128]. Consistent with this, mutations in *MYH6*, a downstream transcriptional target of GATA4 and TBX5, was implicated as a cause of human atrial septal defects. TBX5, GATA4 and NKX2-5 function together only to activate genes. The overlapping expression patterns and complex interactions of these transcription factors allow fine regulation of cardiac gene expression and morphogenesis [20, 129-131] (Figure 2).

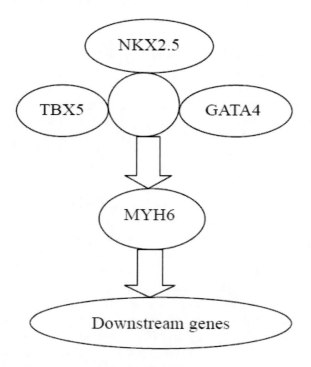

Figure 2. Interaction of NKX2.5, TBX5 and GATA4.

REGULATORY PATHWAY OF CARDIAC GENES

Several types of congenital heart disease involve valve defects of varying severity. Notch signaling is an ancient intercellular signaling mechanism that plays an important role during valve development. Mutations affecting signaling proteins and downstream pathways can lead to valve disease. In mammals, four Notch family receptors have been described: NOTCH1 through to NOTCH4 [20, 132]. The Notch ligands are encoded by the Jagged (*JAG1* and *JAG2*) and Delta-like (*DLL1, DLL3* and *DLL4*) gene families. The Notch signaling pathway is an evolutionarily conserved mechanism used by metazoans to control cell fate decisions through local cell interactions. The notch gene encodes a single-pass transmembrane protein receptor that interacts with its ligands, Delta and Serrate/Jagged. Upon binding of the ligand, the intracellular domain of Notch (NIC) undergoes proteolytic cleavage, and is translocated to the nucleus. In the nucleus, NIC binds to its major downstream effector, Suppressor-of-Hairless (Su(H)). Su(H) binds to the regulatory sequences of the Enhancer-of-Split locus, upregulating the expression of basic helix-loop-helix proteins, which in turn regulate the expression of downstream target genes. Upon ligand binding, a signal is transmitted intracellularly by a process involving the proteolytic cleavage of the receptor and the subsequent nuclear translocation of the Notch intracellular domain (NICD), Figure 3. Alagille syndrome is an autosomal dominant disorder characterized by developmental abnormalities of the liver, heart, eye, skeleton and, at lower penetrance, several other organs. Most cases of Alagille syndrome are caused by *JAG1* mutations, although a small number of Alagille syndrome patients with *NOTCH2* mutations have been identified. The cardiac defects associated with Alagille syndrome include pulmonary artery stenosis and hypoplasia, pulmonic valve stenosis, and tetralogy of Fallot. These defects are likely to be due to a requirement for Notch signaling-mediated differentiation of cardiac neural crest cells into smooth muscle cells, which has been demonstrated in a mouse model. Bicuspid aortic valve affects 1-2% of the population, making it the most common congenital cardiac malformation. Bicuspid aortic valve predisposes one to aortic valve calcification. Aortic valve calcification was linked to Notch regulation of the transcription factor RUNX2. Heterozygous mutations in the *NOTCH1* gene were found in two families with autosomal-dominant aortic valve disease. *NOTCH1* mutations are also found in 4% of sporadic bicuspid aortic valve patients. The formation of bicuspid aortic valve might reflect the role of Notch signaling in regulating the epithelial-mesenchymal transition required for the generation of the heart valves [20, 133, 134]. Recently, mutations in Notch1 in humans have been shown to cause aortic valve defects and activation of Notch1 in mouse leads to abnormal cardiogenesis characterized by deformities of the ventricles and atrioventricular canal. Additionally, mutations in various Notch signaling pathway genes, including Jagged1, mind bomb 1, Hesr1/Hey1, and

Hesr2/Hey2, result in cardiac defects, such as pericardial edema, atrial and ventricular septal defects, cardiac cushion, and valve defects [135-138].

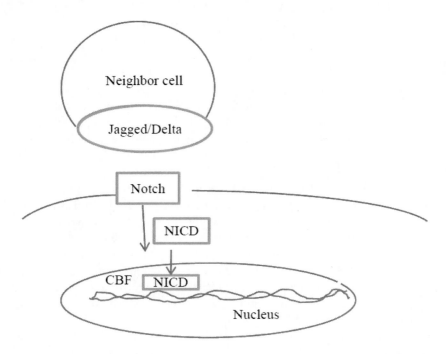

Figure 3. Notch pathway.

MicroRNA Dysfunction

MicroRNAs are natural, single-stranded, non–protein-coding small RNA molecules (~22 nucleotides) that regulate gene expression by binding to target mRNAs and suppress its translation or initiate its degradation. Mature miRNAs are processed from -70 nucleotides long precursor miRNA (pre-miRNAs) that form hairpin secondary structures and that are often evolutionarily conserved. Pre-miRNAs are transcribed from miRNA genes. Although the specific biological roles of most miRNAs are still unknown, functional characterizations of a few of them suggest that these small RNA molecules are involved in many processes of animal development and physiology[139-141]. For example, miR-1 and miR-133 control cardiac and skeletal muscle development [142, 143]. Both genes are under the control of serum response factor, indicating that they are part of a developmental programme regulated by cardiac transcription factors. It has been shown that miR-1 targets the cardiac transcription factor HAND2. Deletion of *miR-1-2* results in heart defects that include VSDs; surviving mice have conduction system defects and increased cardiomyocyte proliferation. Dysregulation of miRNAs might result in congenital heart disease in human [144, 145] (Figure 4).

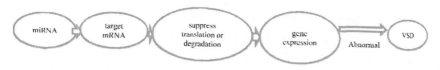

Figure 4. MicroRNAdysfunction results in VSD.

EPIGNETICS

Epigenetics refers to DNA and chromatin modifications that play a critical role in regulation of various genomic functions, and it was then redefined as the study of heritable traits that are not dependent on the primary sequence of DNA. Although the genotype of most cells of a given organism is the same (with the exception of gametes and the cells of the immune system), cellular phenotypes and functions differ radically, and this can be (at least to some extent) controlled by differential epigenetic regulation that is set up during cell differentiation and embryonic morphogenesis [146, 147]. Once the cellular phenotype is established, genomes of somatic cells are 'locked' in tissue-specific patterns of gene expression, generation after generation. This heritability of epigenetic information in somatic cells has been called an 'epigenetic inheritance system' [148]. Even after the epigenomic profiles are established, a substantial degree of epigenetic variation can be generated during the mitotic divisions of a cell in the absence of any specific environmental factors. Such variation is most likely to be the outcome of stochastic events in the somatic inheritance of epigenetic profiles. From the epigenetic point of view, phenotypic differences in monozygous twins could result, in part, from their epigenetic differences. It has recently become clear that epigenetic regulators play crucial roles in the global shaping and maintenance of developmental patterning. This involves dynamic tissue and cell type-specific changes during patterning, as well as the maintenance of the cellular memory that is required for developmental stability. BAF60C (also known as SMARCD3), a subunit of the Swi/Snf-like chromatin-remodelling complex BAF, physically links cardiac transcription factors to the BAF complex. Loss of BAF60C results in severe defects in cardiac morphogenesis and impaired activation of a subset of cardiac genes. The muscle-restricted histone methyltransferase SMYD1 (also known as BOP) is a crucial regulator of cardiac chamber growth and differentiation. Histone deacetylases have mostly been characterized as having an important role in heart hypertrophy and development [20] (Figure 5).

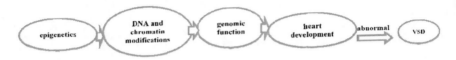

Figure 5. Dysfunctions of epignetics leads to VSD.

STRATEGIES AND FUTURE PERSPECTIVES

The molecular mechanisms of ventricular septal defect are so complex that we have to use diverse strategies to explore them.

Animal Models

Because of the striking homology between mammalian genomes and the many similarities in anatomy, cell biology, and physiology, rat is an excellent animal model for studying of cardiac development and identifying novel genes that could contribute to human disease.

Genome-wide Studies

Recent improvements in genotyping technology and in our knowledge of human genetic variation have made it possible to carry out genome-wide genetic association studies to identify susceptibility genes for common disease. Multistage designs involving large numbers of coding sequence variants (300,000) and relatively large samples sizes (several hundred cases and control subjects) will be essential to reliably detect alleles with appreciable effect sizes

ncrease in relative risk). Direct sequencing of candidate genes in cases
trol subjects provides an alternative approach that can reveal low-
y alleles that influence disease susceptibility [149, 150].

xpression (Microarrays)

)array analysis is a useful tool to obtain a gene expression profile of
wever, current estimates suggest that greater than 60% of human
e more than one isoform. Alternatively, spliced isoforms from the
e can produce proteins with different properties and distinct
The specific roles of gene expression and their splicing variants
'or development need to be further delineated.

A

ulation of miRNAs might result in ventricular septal defect in
rther studies of miRNAs in CHD are required.

's

s increasing evidence that epigenetic modifications, arising
ough DNA methylation and histone modifications may have as
ole as genetics in certain diseases, such as cancer, birth defects,
ul disorders, and psychiatric disorders.

tics

enome project has succeeded, and postgenome era is following.
me comprises 30, 000-40, 000 genes, but their functions,
action, and regulation remain unknown. Bioinformatics is a
indispensable tool in exploring the molecular mechanisms of
2].
:ular basis of ventricular septal defect is an exciting and rapidly
The continuing advances in the understanding of the molecular
f cardiac development will lead to a better understanding of the

genetic basis of ventricular septal defect and hopefully result in improved genetic counseling and care of affected individuals and their families.

ACKNOWLEDGMENTS

This study was supported by the Ruikang Hospital Natural Science Foundation (code: ZKZ201001).

REFERENCES

[1]   Hoffman J. I., KaplanS. The incidence of congenital heart disease, *J Am Coll Cardiol.* 2002;39:1890-1900.

[2]   Garg V. Insights into the genetic basis of congenital heart disease, *Cell Mol. Life Sci.* 2006; 63:1141–1148.

[3]   Kohl H. W. 3rd. Rubella screening and vaccination follow-up by hospital employee health office, *Am J Infect Control.* 1985;13:124-7.

[4]   Singh M., Shah G. L., Singh K. P. Teratogenic effects of dilantin o thoraco-abdominal organs of developing chick embryos, *Indian J Ex Biol.* 2000;38:1026-30.

[5]   Dawson B. V., Johnson P. D., Goldberg S. J. et al. Cardiac teratogenes of halogenated hydrocarbon-contaminated drinking water, *J Am Co Cardiol.* 1993;21:1466-72.

[6]   Kumar S. D., Dheen S. T., Tay S. S. Maternal diabetes induc congenital heart defects in mice by altering the expression of gen involved in cardiovascular development, *Cardiovasc Diabetol.* 2007; 34.

[7]   McCart A., Latchford A., Volikos E. et al. A novel exon duplicati event leading to a truncating germ-line mutation *Fam Canc* 2006;5:205-8.

[8]   Kakavas V. K., Plageras P., Vlachos T. A. et al. PCR-SSCP: a meth for the molecular analysis of genetic diseases. *Mol Biotechnol.* 2008; 155-63.

[9]   Moorman A. F., Christoffels V. M. Cardiac chamber formati development, genes, and evolution. *Physiol Rev.* 2003; 83: 1223–1267

[10] Michael E. Mitchell, Tara L. et al. The molecular basis of congen heart disease. *Semin Thorac Cardiovasc Surg.* 2007; 19:228-237.

[11] Dunwoodie S. L. Combinatorial signaling in the heart orchestrates cardiac induction, lineage specification and chamber formation. *Semin Cell Dev Biol.* 2007;18(1):54-66.

[12] Brand T. Heart development: molecular insights into cardiac specification and early morphogenesis. *Dev Biol.* 2003;258:1–19.

[13] Gruber P. J., Epstein J. A. Epstein. Development gone awry congenital heart disease. *Circ Res.* 2004;94:273-283.

[14] Grego-Bessa J., Luna-Zurita L., del Monte G. et al. Notch signaling is essential for ventricular chamber development. *Dev Cell.* 2007;12:415–429.

[15] Risebro C. A., Riley P. R. Formation of the ventricles. *Scientific World Journal.* 2006;6:1862-80.

[16] Cohen E. D., Tian Y., Morrisey E. E. Wnt signaling: an essential regulator of cardiovascular differentiation, morphogenesis and progenitor self-renewal. *Development.* 2008;135:789-98.

[17] Xiao H., Zhang Y. Y. Understanding the role of transforming growth factor-beta signalling in the heart: overview of studies using genetic mouse models. *Clin Exp Pharmacol Physiol.* 2008;35:335-41.

[18] Moon J. I., Birren S. J. Target-dependent inhibition of sympathetic neuron growth via modulation of a BMP signaling pathway. *Dev Biol.* 2008; 315:404-17.

[19] Mjaatvedt C. H., Nakaoka T., Moreno-Rodriguez R. et al. The outflow tract of the heart is recruited from a novel heart-forming field. *Dev. Biol.* 2001; 238: 97–109.

[20] Bruneau B. G. The developmental genetics *Nature.* 2008; 451:943-8.

[21] High F. A., Epstein J. A. The multifaceted role of Notch in cardiac development and disease. *Nat Rev Genet.* 2008;9:49-61.

[22] Armstrong E. J., Bischoff J. Heart valve development: endothelial cell signaling and differentiation. *Circ Res.* 2004;3;95:459-70.

[23] Yutzey K. E., Colbert M., Robbins J. Ras-related signaling pathways in valve development:ebb and flow. *Physiology* (Bethesda). 2005;20:390-7.

[24] Joziasse I. C., van de Smagt J. J., Smith K. et al. Genes in congenital heart disease: atrioventricular valve formation. *Basic Res Cardiol.* 2008; 103:216-27.

[25] Pierpont M. E., Basson C. T., Benson D. W. et al. Genetic basis for congenital heart defects: current knowledge: a scientific statement from the American Heart Association Congenital Cardiac Defects Committee, Council on Cardiovascular Disease in the Young: endorsed by the American Academy of Pediatrics. *Circulation.* 2007;115:3015–3038.

[26] Ikeda Y., Hiroi Y., Hosoda T. et al. Novel point mutation in the cardiac transcription factor CSX/NKX2.5 associated with congenital heart disease. *Circ J.* 2002;66:561–563.

[27] McElhinney D. B., Geiger E., Blinder J. et al. NKX2.5 mutations in patients with congenital heart disease. *J Am Coll Cardiol.* 2003; 42:1650 –1655.

[28] Elliott D. A., Kirk E. P., Yeoh T. et al. Cardiac homeobox gene NKX2– 5 mutations and congenital heart disease: associations with atrial septal defect and hypoplastic left heart syndrome. *J Am Coll Cardiol.* 2003;41: 2072–2076.

[29] Schubbert S., Zenker M., Rowe S. L. et al. Germline KRAS mutations cause Noonan syndrome. *Nat Genet.* 2006;38:331–336.

[30] Tartaglia M., Kalidas K., Shaw A. et al. PTPN11 mutations in Noonan syndrome: molecular spectrum, genotype-phenotype correlation, and phenotypic heterogeneity. *Am J Hum Genet.* 2002;70:1555–1563.

[31] Yang Y. Q., Wang J., Liu X. Y. et al. Novel GATA4 mutations *Med Sci Monit.* 2012; 18:CR344-50.

[32] Wu G., Shan J., Pang S. et al. Genetic analysis of the promoter *Transl Res.* 2012;159:376-82.

[33] Yamamura N., Kishimoto T. Epigenetic regulation of GATA4 expression by histone *Exp Mol Pathol.* 2012;93:35-9.

[34] He A., Shen X., Ma Q. et al. PRC2 directly methylates GATA4 and represses its transcriptional activity. *Genes Dev.* 2012;26:37-42.

[35] Lee S., Lee J. W., Lee S. K. UTX, a histone *Dev Cell.* 2012;22:25-37.

[36] Risebro C. A., Petchey L. K., Smart N. et al. Epistatic rescue of Nkx2.5 adult cardiac conduction *Circ Res.* 2012;111:e19-31.

[37] Feenstra B., Geller F., Krogh C., Hollegaard M. V. et al. Common variants near MBNL1 and NKX2-5 are associated with infantile hypertrophic pyloric stenosis *Nat Genet.* 2012;44:334-7.

[38] Lee S., Lee J. W., Lee S. K. UTX, a histone *Dev Cell.* 2012;22:25-37.

[39] Wang J., Liu X. Y., Yang Y. Q. Novel NKX2-5 mutations *Genet Mol Res.* 2011;10:2905-15.

[40] Gray R. T., O'Donnell M. E., McGuigan J. A. et al. Quantification of tumour and circulating vascular endothelial growth factor (VEGF) *Br J Biomed Sci.* 2012;69:71-5.

[41] Hu K., Zhang Y., Wang R. et al. Current evidence *Twin Res Hum Genet.* 2012;15:496-502.

[42] Lu K. V., Chang J. P., Parachoniak C. A. et al. VEGF inhibits tumor *Cancer Cell.* 2012;22:21-35.

[43] Sunshine S. B., Dallabrida S. M., Durand E. et al. Endostatin lowers blood *Proc Natl Acad Sci U S A*. 2012;109:11306-11.

[44] Williams E., Martin S., Moss R. et al. Co-expression of VEGF and CA9 in ovarian high-grade serous carcinoma *Virchows Arch*. 2012;461:33-9.

[45] Wu Z. Z., Sun., Chao C. C. Knockdown of CITED2 using short-hairpin RNA *J Cell Physiol*. 2011; 226:2415-28.

[46] Yoshida T., Sekine T., Aisaki K. et al. CITED2 is activated in ulcerative colitis *J Gastroenterol*. 2011;46:339-49.

[47] Lou X., Sun., Chen W. et al. Negative feedback regulation of NF-κB action by CITED2 in the nucleus *J Immunol*. 2011;186:539-48.

[48] Teslovich T. M., Musunuru K., Smith A. V. et al. Biological, clinical and population *Nature*. 2010; 466: 707-13.

[49] Coen K., Flannagan R. S., Baron S. et al. Lysosomal calcium *J Cell Biol*. 2012;198:23-35.

[50] Takeo K., Watanabe N., Tomita T. et al. Contribution of the γ-secretase subunits to the formation *J Biol Chem*. 2012;287:25834-43.

[51] Duncan M. J., Smith J. T., Franklin K. M. et al. Effects of aging and genotype *Exp Neurol*. 2012;236:249-58.

[52] Das H. K., Tchedre K., Mueller B. Repression of transcription *J Neurochem*. 2012;122:487-500.

[53] Moretti J., Chastagner P., Liang C. C. et al. The ubiquitin *J Biol Chem*. 2012; 287: 29429-41.

[54] Afshar Y., Miele L., Fazleabas A. T. Notch1 is regulated by chorionic gonadotropin *Endocrinology*. 2012;153:2884-96.

[55] Krikelis D., Pentheroudakis G., Goussia A. et al. Profiling immunohistochemical expression of NOTCH1-3, JAGGED1, cMET, and phospho-MAPK in 100 carcinomas of unknown primary. *Clin Exp Metastasis*. 2012;29:603-14.

[56] Haydu J. E., de Keersmaecker K., Duff M. K. et al. An activating intragenic deletion in NOTCH1 in human *Blood*. 2012; 119: 5211-4.

[57] Ai Q., Ma X., Huang Q. et al. High-level expression of Notch1 increased the risk *PLoS One*. 2012;7:e35022.

[58] Bergen S. E., O'Dushlaine C. T., Ripke S. et al. Genome-wide association study in a Swedish population *Mol Psychiatry*. 2012;17880-6.

[59] Yang T., Puckerin A., Colecraft H. M. Distinct RGK GTPases *PLoS One*. 2012;7:e37079.

[60] Jangsangthong W., Kuzmenkina E., Böhnke A. K. et al. Single-channel monitoring of reversible L-type Ca(2+) channel Ca(V)α(1)-Ca(V)β subunit interaction. *Biophys J*. 2011;101:2661-70.

[61] Aita Y., Kurebayashi N., Hirose S. et al. Protein kinase D regulates the human *FEBS Lett.* 2011;585:3903-6.

[62] Wang F., McIntosh A. M., He Y. et al. The association of genetic variation in CACNA1C with structure *Bipolar Disord.* 2011;13:696-700.

[63] Goodyer W. R., Gu X., Liu Y. et al. Neonatal β cell development in mice *Dev Cell.* 2012; 23: 21-34.

[64] Hisamitsu T., Nakamura T. Y., Wakabayashi S. Na(+)/H(+) exchanger 1 directly binds to calcineurin A and activates downstream NFAT signaling, leading to cardiomyocyte hypertrophy *Mol Cell Biol.* 2012; 32:3265-80.

[65] Kaminuma O., Kitamura N., Mori A. et al. NFAT1 and NFAT2 differentially regulate IL-17 *Int Arch Allergy Immunol.* 2012;158 Suppl 1:30-4.

[66] le Roy C., Deglesne P. A., Chevallier N., Beitar T., Eclache V., Quettier M., Boubaya M., Letestu R., Lévy V., Ajchenbaum-Cymbalista F, et al. The degree of BCR and NFAT activation predicts clinical outcomes in chronic lymphocytic leukemia *Blood.* 2012;120:356-65.

[67] Close P., East P., Dirac-Svejstrup A. B. et al. DBIRD complex integrates alternative mRNA *Nature.* 2012;484:386-9.

[68] Shi S., Zhou B., Wang Y. et al. Genetic variation in RTN4 3'-UTR and susceptibility *DNA* 2012; 31(6):1088-94.

[69] Li H., Chen Y., Zhou B. et al. RNT4 3'-UTR insertion *DNA* 2012;31:1121-4.

[70] Zhang L., Kuang X., Zhang J. Nogo receptor 3, a paralog of Nogo-66 receptor 1 (NgR1), may function as a NgR1 co-receptor for Nogo-66. *J Genet Genomics.* 2011;38:515-23.

[71] Emanuele M. J., Elia A. E., Xu Q., Thoma C. R. et al. Global identification *Cell.* 2011; 147: 459-74.

[72] Kim W., Bennett E. J., Huttlin E. L. et al. Systematic and quantitative assessment *Mol Cell.* 2011;44:325-40.

[73] Zheng G. F., Wei D., Zhao H. et al. A novel GATA6 mutation *Int J Mol Med.* 2012;29:1065-71.

[74] Lin L., Bass A. J., Lockwood W. W. et al. Activation of GATA binding protein 6 (GATA6) sustains oncogenic lineage-survival *Proc Natl Acad Sci U S A.* 2012;109:4251-6.

[75] Lango Allen H., Flanagan S. E., Shaw-Smith C. et al. International Pancreatic Agenesis Consortium, Ferrer J, Hattersley AT, Ellard S. GATA6 haploinsufficiency causes pancreatic agenesis in humans. *Nat Genet.* 2011;44:20-2.

[76] Cecener G., Tunca B., Egeli U. et al. The promoter *Cell Mol Neurobiol.* 2012;32:237-44.

[77] Wilk J. B., Shrine N. R., Loehr L. R. et al. Genome-Wide Association Studies Identify CHRNA5/3 and HTR4 in the Development of Airflow Obstruction. *Am J Respir Crit Care Med.* 2012;186:622-32.

[78] Fox., Liu Y., White C. C. et al. Genome-wide association for abdominal subcutaneous and visceral adipose *PLoS Genet.* 2012;8:e1002695.

[79] Stevens K. N., Lindstrom S., Scott C. G. et al. Identification of a novel percent mammographic density locus *Hum Mol Genet.* 2012; 21:3299-305.

[80] Hajj H., Dagle J. M. Genetics of patent ductus arteriosus *Semin Perinatol.* 2012;36:98-104.

[81] Yang J., Liao W., Ma Y. Role of SALL4 in hematopoiesis. *Curr Opin Hematol.* 2012;19:287-91.

[82] Trinh D. T., Shibata K., Hirosawa T. et al. Diagnostic utility of CD117, CD133, SALL4, OCT4, TCL1 and glypican-3 in malignant germ cell tumors *J Obstet Gynaecol Res.* 2012;38:841-8.

[83] Yang J., Corsello T. R., Ma Y. Stem cell gene SALL4 suppresses transcription *J Biol Chem.* 2012;287:1996-2005.

[84] Kobayashi D., Kuribayashi K., Tanaka M. et al. Overexpression of SALL4 in lung cancer *Oncol Rep.* 2011;26:965-70.

[85] Jeong H. W., Cui W., Yang Y. et al. SALL4, a stem cell factor, affects the side population *PLoS One.* 2011;6:e18372.

[86] Xu Y. J., Wang J., Xu R. et al. Detecting 22q11.2 deletion in Chinese children *BMC Med Genet.* 2011; 12: 169.

[87] Pereira L. A., Wong M. S., Lim S. M. et al. Brachyury and related Tbx proteins *PLoS One.* 2011;6:e28394.

[88] Guo T., McDonald-McGinn D., Blonska A. et al. Genotype and cardiovascular phenotype *Hum Mutat.* 2011; 32: 1278-89.

[89] van Winkel R; Genetic Risk and Outcome of Psychosis (GROUP) Investigators. Family-based analysis of genetic variation underlying psychosis *Arch Gen Psychiatry.* 2011;68:148-57.

[90] Griffin H. R., Töpf A., Glen E. et al. Systematic survey of variants in TBX1 in non-syndromic tetralogy *Heart.* 2010;96:1651-5.

[91] Zhang Q., Yu D., Seo S., Stone E. M. et al. Intrinsic protein-protein interaction-mediated and chaperonin-assisted sequential assembly of stable bardet-biedl syndrome *J Biol Chem.* 2012;287:20625-35.

[92] Marion V., Schlicht D., Mockel A., Caillard S. et al. Bardet-Biedl syndrome *Kidney Int.* 2011;79:1013-25.

[93] Booij J. C., Bakker A., Kulumbetova J. et al. Simultaneous mutation *Ophthalmology.* 2011;118: 160-167.e1-3.

[94] Bailey S. D., Xie C., Do R. et al. Variation at the NFATC2 locus *Diabetes Care.* 2010;33:2250-3.

[95] Billingsley G., Bin J., Fieggen K. J. et al. Mutations in chaperonin-like BBS genes *J Med Genet.* 2010;47:453-63.

[96] Gong M., Chen Y., Senturia R. et al. Caspases cleave and inhibit the microRNA *Protein Sci.* 2012;21:797-808.

[97] Barr I., Smith A. T., Chen Y. et al. Ferric, not ferrous, heme *Proc Natl Acad Sci USA* 2012;109:1919-24.

[98] Wada T., Kikuchi J., Furukawa Y. Histone deacetylase 1 enhances microRNA *EMBO Rep.* 2012; 13:142-9.

[99] Barr I., Smith A. T., Senturia R. et al. DiGeorge critical region 8 (DGCR8) is a double-cysteine *J Biol Chem.* 2011; 286:16716-25.

[100] Bennett E. J., Rush J., Gygi S. P. et al. Dynamics of cullin-RING ubiquitin *Cell.* 2010;143:951-65.

[101] Lindskog C., Korsgren O., Pontén F. et al. Novel pancreatic beta cell-specific proteins *J Proteomics.* 2012;75:2611-20.

[102] Xu B., Roos J. L., Dexheimer P. et al. Exome sequencing *Nat Genet.* 2011;43:864-8.

[103] Wang P., Yu P., Gao P. et al. Discovery of novel human BMC Genomics. *BMC Genomics.* 2009;10:518.

[104] Vinayagam A., Stelzl U., Foulle R. et al. A directed protein interaction network for investigating intracellular signal transduction *Sci Signal.* 2011;4:rs8.

[105] Wagner S. A., Beli P., Weinert B. T. et al. A proteome *Mol Cell Proteomics.* 2011;10:M111.013284.

[106] Talmud P. J., Drenos F., Shah S. et al. Gene-centric association signals *Am J Hum Genet.* 2009;85:628-42.

[107] Barbe L., Lundberg E., Oksvold P. et al. Andersson-Svahn H. Toward a confocal subcellular atlas of the human *Mol Cell Proteomics.* 2008;7:499-508.

[108] Saus E., Brunet A., Armengol L. et al. Comprehensive copy number variant (CNV) analysis of neuronal pathways *J Psychiatr Res.* 2010; 44:971-8.

[109] Pfuhl T., Dürr M., Spurk A. et al. Biochemical characterisation of the proteins encoded by the DiGeorge critical region 6 (DGCR6) genes. *Hum Genet.* 2005;117:70-80.

[110] Pfuhl T., Dürr M., Spurk A. et al. Biochemical characterisation of the proteins *Hum Genet.* 2005;117:70-80.

[111] Gerhard D. S., Wagner L., Feingold E. A. et al. The status, quality, and expansion of the NIH full-length cDNA *Genome Res.* 2004;14:2121-7.

[112] Nguyen H. H., Takata R., Akamatsu S. et al. IRX4 at 5p15 suppresses prostate cancer *Hum Mol Genet.* 2012; 21: 2076-85.

[113] Kim W., Bennett E. J., Huttlin E. L. et al. Systematic and quantitative assessment *Mol Cell.* 2011;44(2): 325-40.

[114] Schürks M., Buring J. E., Ridker P. M. et al. Genetic determinants of cardiovascular events among women with migraine: a genome *PLoS One.* 2011;6:e22106.

[115] Cheng Z., Wang J., Su D. et al. Two novel mutations *Hum Genet.* 2011;130:657-62.

[116] Bailey S. D., Xie C., Do R. et al. DREAM investigators. Variation at the NFATC2 locus *Diabetes Care.* 2010;33:2250-3.

[117] Kawame H., Adachi M., Tachibana K. et al. Graves' disease in patients with 22q11.2 deletion. *J Pediatr.* 2001;139:892-5.

[118] Jawad A. F., McDonald-Mcginn D. M., Zackai E. et al. Immunologic features of chromosome *J Pediatr.* 2001;139:715-23.

[119] Driscoll D. A., Spinner N. B., Budarf M. L. et al. Deletions and microdeletions of 22q11.2 in velo-cardio-facial syndrome *Am J Med Genet.* 1992;44:261-8.

[120] Clark E. B. *Mechanisms in the pathogenesis of congenital heart disease.* In: Pierpont M. E., Moller J., editors. The genetics of cardiovascular disease. Boston, MA' Martinus-Nijoff; 1986. p. 3 –11.

[121] Clark E. B. Pathogenetic mechanisms of congenital cardiovascular malformations revisited. *Semin Perinatol* 1996;20:465– 72.

[122] Benoit G. Bruneau. The developmental genetics of congenital heart disease. *Nature.* 2008;451:943-8.

[123] Hyun C., Lavulo L. Congenital heart diseases in small animals: Part I. Genetic pathways and potential candidate genes. *The Veterinary Journal;* 2006; 171: 245–255.

[124] Hiroi, Kudoh, Monzen K. et al. Tbx5 associates with Nkx2-5 and synergistically promotes cardiomyocyte differentiation. *Nat. Genet.* 2001;28: 276–280.

[125] Goldmuntz, Geiger, Benson D. W. NKX2.5 mutations in patients with tetralogy of fallot. *Circulation.* 2001; 104: 2565–2568.

[126] Stennard F. A., Costa M. W., Elliott D. A. et al. Cardiac T-box factor Tbx20 directly interacts with Nkx2-5, GATA4, and GATA5 in

regulation of gene expression in the developing heart. *Dev Biol.* 2003; 262:206-24.

[127] Pashmforoush M., Lu J. T., Chen H. et al. Nkx2-5 pathways and congenital heart disease: loss of ventricular myocyte lineage specification leads to progressive cardiomyopathy and complete heart block. *Cell.* 2004; 117: 373–386.

[128] Pu W. T., Ishiwata T., Juraszek A. L. et al. GATA4 is a dosage-sensitive regulator of cardiac morphogenesis. *Dev. Biol.* 2004; 275: 235–244.

[129] Moskowitz I. P., Kim J. B., Moore M. L. et al. A molecular pathway including Id2, Tbx5, and Nkx2-5 required for cardiac conduction system development. *Cell.* 2007;129:1365-76.

[130] Ching Y. H., Ghosh T. K., Cross S. J. et al. Mutation in myosin heavy chain 6 causes atrial septal defect. *Nat. Genet.* 2005;37: 423–428.

[131] Varadkar P., Kraman M., Despres D. et al. Notch2 is required for the proliferation of cardiac neural crest-derived smooth muscle cells. *Dev Dyn.* 2008;237:1144-52.

[132] del Monte G., Grego-Bessa J., González-Rajal A. et al. Monitoring Notch1 activity in development: evidence for a feedback regulatory loop. *Dev Dyn.* 2007;236:2594-614.

[133] Kwon C., Arnold J., Hsiao E. C. et al. Canonical Wnt signaling is a positive regulator of mammalian cardiac progenitors. *Proc Natl Acad Sci USA.* 2007;104:10894-9.

[134] Miller C. T., Swartz M. E., Khuu P. A. et al. mef2ca is required in cranial neural crest to effect Endothelin1 signaling in zebrafish. *Dev Biol.* 2007;308:144-57.

[135] Ren X., Li Y., Ma X. et al. Activation of p38/MEF2C pathway by all-trans retinoic acid in cardiac myoblasts. *Life Sci.* 2007;81:89-96.

[136] Ueno S., Weidinger G., Osugi T. et al. Biphasic role for Wnt/beta-catenin signaling in cardiac specification in zebrafish and embryonic stem cells. *Proc Natl Acad Sci USA.* 2007;104:9685-90.

[137] Groenendijk B. C., Stekelenburg-de Vos S., Vennemann P. et al. The endothelin-1 pathway and the development of cardiovascular defects in the haemodynamically challenged chicken embryo. *J Vasc Res.* 2008; 45:54-68.

[138] Couzin J. Breakthrough of The Year: Small RNAs make big splash, *Science.* 2002, 298:2296-2297.

[139] Liu C. G., Calin G. A., Meloon B. et al. An oligonucleotide microchip for genome-wide microRNA profiling in human and mouse tissues. *Proc Natl Acad Sci USA.* 2004;101:9740-4.

[140] Lee C. T., Risom T., Strauss W. M. MicroRNAs in mammalian development. *Birth Defects Res C Embryo Today.* 2006, 78:129-139.

[141] Zhang B., Wang Q., Pan X. MicroRNAs and their regulatory roles in animals and plants, *J Cell Physiol.* 2007, 210: 279-289.

[142] Zhao Y. Ransom J. F., Li A. et al. Dysregulation of cardiogenesis, cardiac conduction, and cell cycle in mice lacking miRNA-1-2. *Cell.* 2007; 129:303–317.

[143] Zhao Y., Samal E., Srivastava D. Serum sponse factor regulates a muscle-specific microRNA that targets Hand2 during cardiogenesis, *Nature.* 2005, 436:214-220.

[144] Kwon C., Han Z., Olson E. N. et al. MicroRNA1 influences cardiac differentiation in Drosophila and regulates Notch signaling, *Proc Natl Acad Sci USA.* 2005, 102:18986–18991.

[145] Wong A. H., Gottesman I. I., Petronis A. Phenotypic differences in genetically identical organisms: the epigenetic perspective. *Human Molecular Genetics,* 2005, 14:R11–R18.

[146] Armstrong L., Lako M., Dean W. et al. Epigenetic modification is central to genome reprogramming in somatic cell nuclear transfer. *Stem Cells.* 2006; 24:805-814.

[147] Jacinto F. V., Esteller M., Mutator pathways unleashed by epigenetic silencing in human cancer. *Mutagenesis.* 2007;22:247-53.

[148] Cohen J. C. Genetic approaches to coronary heart disease. *J Am Coll Cardiol.* 2006;48:A10–A14.

[149] Wallace C., Newhouse S. J., Braund P. et al. Genomewide association study identifies genes for biomarkers of cardiovascular disease: serum urate and dyslipidemia. *Am J Hum Genet.* 2008; 82:139–149.

[150] Todd A. K. Bioinformatics approaches to quadruplex sequence location. *Methods.* 2007;43:246–251.

[151] Yang W., Paschen W. Conditional gene silencing in mammalian cells mediated by a stress-inducible promoter. *Biochem Biophys Res Commun.* 2008;365:521-7.

In: Atrial and Ventricular Septal Defects   ISBN: 978-1-62618-326-1
Editor: Steven A. Larkin   © 2013 Nova Science Publishers, Inc.

Chapter 2

MATERNAL CHARACTERISTICS AND USE OF DRUGS AND SEPTUM HEART DEFECTS IN THE CHILD: A POPULATION-BASED STUDY

Bengt Källén [*]

Tornblad Institute, University of Lund, Lund, Sweden

ABSTRACT

Congenital cardiac septum defects are common malformations. A large number of possible causal factors have been published, mainly from retrospective case-control studies. The present analysis is based on Swedish health registers and investigates some maternal risk factors for ventricular (VSD) and atrial (ASD) septum defects. A total of 7308 children with septum defects were identified with the use of three different national registers and risk factors were ascertained from the Medical Birth Register and consist of data collected in early pregnancy.

Maternal age and parity have weak effects on the risk for septum defects, similar for VSD and ASD. Maternal smoking in early pregnancy was associated with an increased risk for ASD but a slightly decreased risk for VSD. Maternal overweight or obesity was associated with an

---

[*] Corresponding author: Professor Bengt Källén, Tornblad Institute, Biskopsgatan 7, SE 232 62 Lund, Sweden. Tel: 046-46-222 7536, Fax: +46-46-222 4226. E-mail: Bengt.Kallen@ med.lu.se.

increased risk for ASD but not for VSD. Couple subfertility (evaluated from number of years of unwanted childlessness) was a stronger risk factor for ASD than for VSD. Maternal pre-existing diabetes (mainly type 1) was a strong factor with a three times increased risk for any septum defect, highest for combined VSD+ASD, intermediate for only ASD, and lowest for only VSD.

Children with a septum defect were born preterm more often than other children and the highest odds ratio for preterm birth was seen for ASD. There was an excess of females, most pronounced for combined VSD+ASD. There was an excess of multiple births, notably for ASD.

Maternal use of a wide spectrum of drugs was analyzed with adjustments made for year of birth, maternal age, parity, smoking, and BMI. Increased risks were seen for a number of drug categories. Use of aminosalicylic acid drugs was associated with an increased risk (OR = 1.76) and also use of immunosuppressive drugs (OR = 3.31), both may at least partly be due to underlying pathology. This is probably the case also for the increased risk after use of thyroxin (OR = 1.22). An increased risk was also seen after antihypertensive drugs (OR = 1.61), anticonvulsants (OR = 1.74), tricyclic antidepressants (OR = 1.95) and paroxetine (OR = 2.15). No effect was seen for other antidepressants or from NSAIDs (including ibuprofen). An increased risk after use of vitamin B12 could be explained by concomitant drug use.

To conclude, some maternal characteristics and chronic diseases were risk factors for cardiac septum defects in the child and the maternal use of a few drugs may also carry a risk.

Keywords: Diabetes, obesity, drug use, ventricular septum defect, atrium septum defect, epidemiology

INTRODUCTION

Cardiovascular defects make up a substantial part of all human congenital malformations. The total rate of congenital malformations in newborns depends on the inclusion criteria applied and the length of the follow-up time of the children. The same is true for cardiovascular defects which sometimes are not diagnosed until after the neonatal period. A rough estimate is that one per cent of all newborns have a congenital heart defect, the severity of which varies from lethal conditions to mild anomalies which allow a normal life. A large part of the cardiovascular defects consists of ventricular (VSD) or atrial (ASD) septum defects with an occurrence of approximately 0.5-0.6 per cent. Also in this group of defects, the severity varies. Among infants with VSD, some have membranous defects, other muscular defects. Some of the latter may close spontaneously. There are two basic types of atrial septum defects, primary and secondary septum defects. A morphologically open foramen ovale is a common condition which normally causes no anomaly of cardiac function and should not be included among atrial septum defects.

Numerous studies have been published on etiological factors involved in the formation of cardiovascular malformations, including septum defects. Many of the largest studies were retrospective case-control studies with exposure information obtained from maternal interviews or questionnaires [1-4]. These studies carry a risk of recall bias and some of them also have a problem with a high rate of non-responders. Other studies are cohort studies, analyzing the occurrence of such defects in a defined cohort of women with a certain exposure, often of limited size and sometimes with low statistical power. Studies based on various health registers have contributed information based on large numbers and exposure data obtained prospectively in relation to the outcome (e.g., [5]).

A review of some of the relevant literature was published in 2007 [6]. Only few drugs were definitely linked to an increased risk for cardiovascular defects. Except for the well-known teratogens thalidomide and isotretinoin, only ibuprofen was thought to be linked to septum defects. A long list was given of drugs where data were insufficient to determine risks for cardiovascular defects. Since this paper was published, the possibility that antihypertensive drugs could increase the risk for septum defects has been raised, both in a retrospective case-control study [4] and in a large register study [7]. Another group of drugs which has been much discussed is antidepressants, notably selective serotonin reuptake inhibitor (SSRI) drugs, where some studies found an increased risk for cardiovascular malformations after any SSRI drug [8, 9] while other studies found no general harmful effect of SSRI drugs but an increased risk after the use of paroxetine [10].

The present study used Swedish health registers in an analysis of some risk factors for cardiac septum defects with special reference to the impact of maternal disease and drug use in early pregnancy.

MATERIAL AND METHODS

Children with a diagnosis of VSD or ASD (or both) and born between January 1, 1998 and December 31, 2010 were identified from three sources [11]. 1) The Swedish Medical Birth Register (MBR) [12] which contains medical information on nearly all deliveries in Sweden, including diagnoses given at the pediatric examination which every infant gets by a qualified pediatrician soon after birth. 2) The Swedish Register of Congenital Malformations (RCM) (also called the Birth Defect Register) which is based on compulsory reporting of major malformations to the National Board of Health and Welfare, mainly from pediatricians but also from other specialists, including child cardiologists. 3) The Hospital Discharge Register (HDR) which is based on inpatient discharge diagnoses from all hospitals in Sweden. In all three registers, malformation diagnoses were recorded as International Classification of Diseases (ICD) -10 codes and patient identification with the unique 12-digit identification number every person living in Sweden has.

Using these sources, a file was formed including each child with one or both of the septum defect diagnoses, the source(s) of ascertainment, and with information on the pregnancy and delivery obtained from the MBR. Children who had immigrated after birth were thus not included. The file contained children who had no code indicating a chromosomal anomaly (Q9) and who had no other cardiovascular diagnoses than VSD (Q21.0) or ASD (Q21.1), or both. Only patent ductus (Q25.0), single umbilical artery (Q27.0), and unspecified cardiac defect (Q24.9) were allowed together with the septum defect diagnoses.

For all children (with or without septum defects) maternal and some infant characteristics were obtained from MBR: year of birth, maternal age in 5-year group(<20, 20-24 etc. up to ≥40 years), parity (1, 2, 3, ≥4, where parity 1 means the first infant born by the woman), maternal smoking in early pregnancy (unknown, none, <10 cigarettes per day, ≥10 cigarettes per day), prepregnancy BMI, obtained from reported prepregnancy weight and height (unknown, <19.8, 19.8-24.9, 25-29.9, 30-39.9, ≥40), period of unwanted childlessness (number of years), and information on maternal pre-existing diabetes (ICD codes E10-E14 or O24.0-O24.3).

Information on maternal drug use during early pregnancy was obtained from midwife interviews at the first antenatal care visit, usually during weeks 10-12. The information was recorded in clear text on a standardized form, used all over the country, and the drug names were centrally translated to Anatomic, Therapeutic, Chemical (ATC) codes. Information on exact timing of drug use and the amount used were often incomplete or lacking.

For the infants, information of preterm birth (<37 weeks, mainly based on second trimester ultrasound), sex, and number on infants in the birth were obtained from MBR. The presence of other congenital malformations than septum defects were also recorded, registered with ICD-10 codes. Such malformations were divided into major and minor malformations according to their significance for the child. Information on the malformations was obtained from the same sources as the information on septum defects (MBR, RCM and HDR).

Maternal and infant characteristics among children with septum defects (cases) were compared with all children without such defects (controls) with odds ratios (OR) obtained from Mantel-Haenszel analyses after adjustment for year of birth, maternal age, parity, smoking, and BMI. Using Miettinen´s method, approximate 95% confidence intervals (95% CI) were calculated. Two ORs were compared based on the Mantel-Haenszel variances. When the expected number of exposed cases was low (<10), risk ratios (RR) were calculated instead as observed over expected numbers, and 95% CIs were estimated from exact Poisson distributions. Analyses of drug use were either made for groups of drugs or for specific drugs.

Table 1. Distribution of children with cardiac septum defects according to type and source of information

Septum defect	Only MBR	MBR +RCM	MBR +HDR	Only RCM	RCM +HDR	Only HDR	MBR+RCM + HDR	Total	%
VSD	1669	1489	472	395	104	277	487	4893	67.0
ASD	305	229	212	78	49	387	219	1476	20.2
VSD+ASD	114	295	119	65	53	79	214	939	12.8
Total	2095	2016	803	538	206	743	920	7308	
%	28.7	27.6	11.0	7.4	2.8	10.2	12.6		

HDR = Hospital Discharge Register; MBR = Medical Birth Register; RCM = Register of Congenital Malformations.

RESULTS

A total of 7 308 infants were identified with VSD and/or ASD. Two thirds of them had only VSD, 20% had only ASD and 13% had both VSD and ASD (Table 1). This table also shows the contribution of the various registers to the identification of the cases. Seventy-five per cent of all cases were identified from MBR, 48% were reported to the RCM, and 37% were identified from

HDR. It should be noted that the routines for reporting to RCM were changed in 1999. Before that year heart defects were not supposed to be reported to RCM if not associated with heart failure or cyanosis, but some doctors reported VSD and ASD anyway. Such cases were recorded but excluded from the surveillance of cardiovascular defects but were included in the present study. Table 2 summarizes maternal characteristics. There is a weak increased risk of a septum defect at maternal age of 35 years or higher. As seen in Figure 1, no marked difference is seen between the maternal age dependency of VSD or ASD. The septum defect risk is a little higher at first parity than at higher parities; again no definite difference is seen between VSD and ASD (Figure 2). There is no effect of maternal smoking on the total material but as seen in Figure 3, the two main groups differ. For VSD the risk decreases, for ASD it increases. For the total material there is a faint increase in risk at overweight or obesity. When broken up into VSD and ASD, only the latter shows an increase (Figure 4). There is an excess of subfertility problems among mothers of children with septum defects, evident as an increased risk of having at least a one year period of unwanted childlessness. The excess of three or more years of childlessness is only statistically significant for ASD (OR = 1.69, 95% CI 1.33-2.16). For VSD the OR is 1.17 (95% CI 0.99-1.36) and for VSD+ASD 1.20 (95% CI 0.86-1.69). The difference between VSD and ASD is hardly random (p=0.02). Maternal pre-existing diabetes is a clear-cut risk factor for a septum defect. When analyzed after type of septum defect, the OR was highest for the combined VSD+ASD (OR = 4.28, 95% CI 2.87-6.34), intermediate for only ASD (OR = 3.51, 95% CI 2.46-5.00), and lowest for only VSD (OR =2.57, 95% CI 2.02-3.27). The difference between the OR for only VSD and for VSD+ASD is statistically significant (p=0.04). Table 3 presents some data on the infants. Infants with septum defects were born preterm more often than other infants and this was more marked for ASD than for VSD or VSD+ASD. There is an excess of females, statistically significant only for VSD. There is also an excess of multiple births, strongest for ASD. In only eight twin pairs, both children had a septum defect diagnosis.

Table 2. Maternal characteristics when at least one child had a septum defect

Variable	Child with septum defect	All women	OR	95% CI	Adjusted for
Maternal age					Year of delivery, parity, smoking, BMI
<20	147	22468	1.15	0.97-1.37	
20-24	954	164861	1.01	0.93-1.09	
25-29	2214	309110	1.00	Reference	
30-34	2478	439284	1.05	0.98-1.18	
35-39	1215	207449	**1.33**	**1.16-1.52**	
≥40	292	40613	**1.33**	**1.17-1.52**	
Parity					Year of delivery, age, smoking, BMI
1	3410	564520	1.00	Reference	
2	2494	455149	**0.91**	**0.86-0.96**	
3	952	169841	**0.90**	**0.83-0.98**	
≥4	444	74275	0.93	0.83-1.04	
Smoking					Year of delivery, age, parity, BMI
Unknown	549	83152	-	-	
None	6158	1072755	1.00	Reference	
<10 cigs/day	429	78334	0.95	0.86-1.05	
≥10 cigs/day	164	29544	0.96	0.82-1.13	
BMI					Year of delivery, age, parity, smoking
Unknown	965	158678	-	-	
<19.8	520	94544	0.98	0.89-1.07	
19.8-24.9	3431	612470	1.00	Reference	
25-29.9	1628	275253	**1.06**	**1.00-1.12**	
30-39.9	689	113714	**1.08**	**1.00-1.18**	
≥40	67	9226	**1.28**	**1.00-1.64**	
Unwanted childlessness					Year of delivery, age, parity, smoking, BMI
Any length	639	96989	**1.13**	**1.04-1.23**	
At least 3 years	284	37528	**1.28**	**1.13-1.44**	
Maternal pre-existing diabetes	113	6544	**3.02**	**2.52-3.61**	Year of delivery, age, parity, smoking, BMI
Total	7300	1263785	-	-	-

Odds ratios (OR) with 95% confidence intervals (95% CI), adjusted as marked.
Bold Figures mark statistical significance (p<0.05)

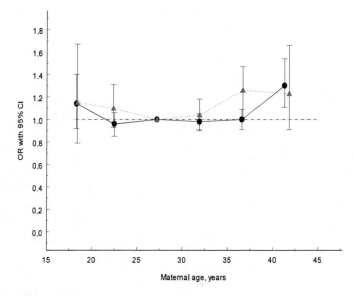

Figure 1. Odds ratio for a septum defect in the child according to maternal age. Unbroken line ventricular septum defect, dotted line atrial septum defect. Vertical lines show 95% confidence intervals. Horizontal dashed line shows reference (OR =1.0).

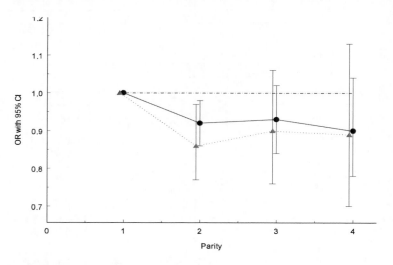

Figure 2. Odds ratio for a septum defect in the child according to parity. Unbroken line ventricular septum defect, dotted line atrial septum defect. Vertical lines show 95% confidence intervals. Horizontal dashed line shows reference (OR =1.0).

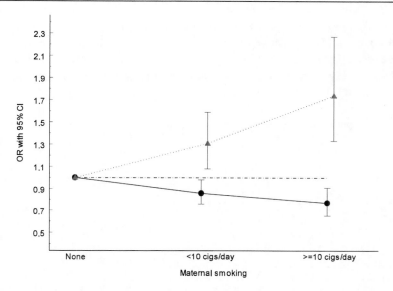

Figure 3. Odds ratio for a septum defect in the child according to maternal smoking in early pregnancy. Unbroken line ventricular septum defect, dotted line atrial septum defect. Vertical lines show 95% confidence intervals. Horizontal dashed line shows reference (OR =1.0).

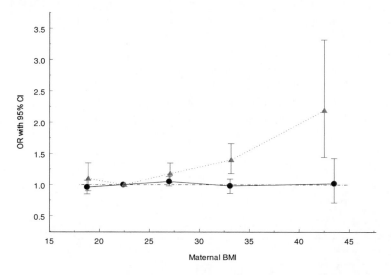

Figure 4. Odds ratio for a septum defect in the child according to maternal BMI. Unbroken line ventricular septum defect, dotted line atrial septum defect. Vertical lines show 95% confidence intervals. Horizontal dashed line shows reference (OR =1.0).

Table 3. Some infant characteristics in the presence of a septum defect. Number of children with septum defects = 7 308, total number of children in population = 1 282 858. Odds ratio (OR) with 95% confidence intervals (95% CI), adjusted for year of birth, maternal age, parity, smoking, and BMI. Bold Figures mark statistical significance (p<0.05)

Variable	Septum defect	Children with septum defect with variable	All children with septum defect[*]	All children with variable	All children[*]	OR	95% CI
Preterm birth	All	1241	7298	34406	1281468	**3.10**	**2.92-3.29**
	VSD	597	4887			**2.11**	**1.94-2.29**
	ASD	494	1473			**7.48**	**6.79-8.23**
	VSD+ASD	150	938			**2.84**	**2.40-3.37**
Male sex	All	3519	7308	659657	1282522	**0.88**	**0.84-0.92**
	VSD	2381	4893			**0.89**	**0.84-0.95**
	ASD	747	1476			0.96	0.87-1.07
	VSD+ASD	391	939			**0.67**	**0.59-0.87**
Multiple birth	All	393	7308	37910	1282858	**1.92**	**1.73-2.12**
	VSD	218	4893			**1.59**	**1.39-1.42**
	ASD	128	1476			**2.90**	**2.42-3.47**
	VSD+ASD	55	939			**2.04**	**1.57-2.66**

[*] Numbers for all children refer to children with information on the variable.
ASD= atrial septum defect, VSD = ventricular septum defect.

Table 4. Comparison of the effect of some maternal characteristics on the risk of a septum defect, including and excluding cases only reported in MBR

	All defects		Defects only reported to MBR excluded	
Variable	OR	95% CI	OR	95% CI
Maternal age 35-39 years	1.33	1.16-1.52	1.38	1.18-1.61
Maternal age ≥40 years	1.33	1.17-1.52	1.39	1.20-1.62
Parity 2	0.91	0.86-0.96	0.92	0.88-0.98
Parity 3	0.90	0.83-0.98	0.90	0.83-0.99
BMI 25-29.9	1.06	1.00-1.12	1.07	1.01-1.15
BMI 30-39.9	1.08	1.00-1.18	1.11	1.01-1.22
BMI ≥40	1.28	1.00-1.86	1.32	1.00-1.74

Table 5. Effect of maternal use of some main drug groups on the risk for a septum defect in the child. Number of children with septum defects = 7 308, total number of children in population = 1 282 858. Odds ratio (OR) with 95% confidence intervals (95% CI), adjusted for year of birth, maternal age, parity, smoking, and BMI. Bold Figures mark statistical significance (p<0.05)

Drug group	No. of exposed infants with septum defects	No. of exposed infants in population	OR	95% CI
H2-antagonists	9	1563	1.07	0.56-2.08
Proton pump inhibitors	33	5856	0.96	0.68-1.35
Aminosalicylic acid drugs	22	2268	**1.76**	**1.18-2.67**
Folic acid	315	55037	0.99	0.88-1.11
Vitamin B12	36	4423	**1.43**	**1.02-1.96**
Antihypertensives	37	3783	**1.61**	**1.17-2.22**
Oral contraceptives	15	2779	0.96	0.56-1.60
Gestagens	35	4656	1.23	0.88-1.71
Ovulation stimulators	16	1798	1.52	0.92-2.51
Systemic glucocorticoids	22	3310	1.17	0.77-1.87
Thyroid hormones	108	15324	**1.22**	**1.00-1.47**
Antibiotics	155	26313	1.05	0.90-1.23
Immunosuppressive drugs	13	719	**3.31**	**1.76-5.56**
NSAIDs	100	15953	1.08	0.89-1.32
Opioids	32	5010	1.12	0.78-1.17
Mild analgesics	407	68954	1.04	0.96-1.15
Drugs for migraine	16	2421	1.13	0.69-1.85
Anticonvulsants	28	2753	**1.74**	**1.31-2.51**
Neuroleptics	18	2732	1.13	0.71-1.79
Sedatives/hypnotics	29	4467	1.13	0.78-1.63
Antidepressants	99	15132	1.13	0.92-1.38
Drugs for rhinitis	69	11600	1.06	0.83-1.34
Antiasthmatics	179	28034	1.12	0.96-1.36
Cough drugs	26	4149	1.11	0.75-1.63
Antihistamines	295	55347	0.94	0.84-1.06

Among the children with VSD, 6.6% had another major congenital malformation while among children with ASD this percentage was 14.2 and among children with both VSD and ASD, it was 10.3. These three proportions differ significantly ($\chi^2_{2 \text{ d.f.}}$ = 85.2, p<0.001). The rate of minor congenital malformations was 2.9% among children with VSD, 3.5% among children with ASD, and 2.4% among children with both VSD and ASD. These three proportions do not differ significantly ($\chi^2_{2.df.}$ = 2.13, p=0.34). Table 4 compares the effect of maternal factors which appeared as significantly associated with the risk of a septum defect when analyzed in the total material and after cases only reported to MBR were removed. In this analysis, the OR estimates are slightly higher than in the original analysis but the differences are small and do not motivate exclusion of cases only reported to MBR. Maternal use of various drugs in early pregnancy and the risk for a septum defect is shown in Table 5. Twenty-five different drugs or drug groups are listed. Among them six show a statistically significantly increased OR. Table 6 eliminates the effect of concomitant use of each of these other drugs and of maternal diabetes. These drug groups, some other groups where the OR estimate either is high or the lower confidence limit is over 0.90, and some drugs which have been discussed in the literature will be further analyzed.

Table 6. Comparison of data from Table 5 with similar data when women who had reported the use of any of the other tabulated drugs or had diabetes were excluded. In this Table are also included vitamin B12, folic acid, and the two antidepressants with significant effects in Table 8. Bold Figures mark statistical significance (p<0.05)

Drug	No. of exposed children	OR	95% CI	No. of exposed children	OR /RR	95% CI
Aminosalicylic acid drugs	22	1.76	1.18-2.67	16	1.46	0.89-2.38
Antihypertensives	37	1.61	1.17-2.22	21	1.19	0.77-1.82
Thyroid hormone	108	1.22	1.00-1.47	96	1.15	0.94-1.71
Immunosuppressive drugs	13	3.31	1.76-5.56	5	1.99	0.65-4.65#
Anticonvulsants	28	1.74	1.31-2.51	22	1.46	0.96-2.21
Tricyclic antidepressant	14	1.95	1.16-3.27	12	1.86	0.96-3.25#
Paroxetine	14	2.15	1.18-3.61	12	**2.02**	**1.04-3.53#**
Vitamin B12	36	1.43	1.02-1.96	24	1.14	0.76-1.70
Folic acid	315	0.99	0.88-1.11	272	0.92	0.81-1.04

Risk ratio (RR) as observed over expected number with exact 95% CI.

Aminosalicylic Acid Drugs

The two main drugs were salazopyrin and mesalazin. Both showed similar RRs for any septum defect (1.68 and 1.72, respectively). The RR for any aminosalicylic acid drug for VSD was 1.31 (95% CI 0.65-2.35), for ASD 2.48 (95% CI 0.91-5.40), and for VSD+ASD 2.02 (95% CI 0.92-6.59). Even though none of these three estimates reached statistical significance, the risk may be higher for ASD (also when combined with VSD) than with VSD but the difference can be random. Only two of the exposed children had another major congenital malformation (1.0 expected from the general rate of other major malformations among infants with septum defects). When women with concomitant drug use or diabetes were removed from the analysis, the estimated OR declined somewhat (Table 6) and lost statistical significance. Among the 22 exposed children with septum defects, six were excluded.

Table 7. Effect of maternal use of antihypertensive drugs on the risk for a septum defect in the child according to type of drug. Number of children with septum defects = 7 308, total number of children in population = 1 282 858. Odds ratio (OR) with 95% confidence intervals (95% CI), adjusted for year of birth, maternal age, parity, smoking, and BMI. Bold Figures mark statistical significance (p<0.05)

Antihypertensive Drug group	Type of septum defect	No. of exposed infants with septum defects	No of exposed infants in population	OR/RR	95% CI
All	All	37	3783	**1.61**	**1.17-2.23**
	VSD	16		1.10	0.66-1.80
	ASD	14		**2.67**	**1.46-4.48#**
	VSD+ASD	7		2.11	0.85-4.36*
Beta-blockers	All	23	2981	1.31	0.86-1.99
	VSD	10		0.87	0.46-1.64
	ASD	12		**1.27**	**1.10-5.62**
	VSD+ASD	1		-	
ACE inhibitors or angiotensin II inhibitors	All	6	1878	**4.32**	**1.18-9.40#**
Other anti-hypertensives	All	20	1123	**2.95**	**1.81-4.56#**
	VSD	7		1.62	0.65-3.35#
	ASD	7		**4.43**	**1.98-10.2#**
	VSD+ASD	6		**5.83**	**2.14-12.7#**

Risk ratio (RR) as observed over expected number with exact 95% CI.

Vitamin B12 and Folic Acid

There is a statistically significant increased risk for any septum defect after maternal use of vitamin B12. It is not significantly increased for VSD (OR = 1.14, 95% CI 0.72-1.79) but is for ASD (OR = 2.25, 95% CI 1.29-1.92) while for combined VSD+ASD the OR estimate is 1.93 (95% CI 0.60-3.45), thus not statistically significant. Only two of the exposed children had another major congenital malformation (2.3 expected). In 12 among the 36 septum defect cases the analysis was complicated by the presence of maternal diabetes or the concomitant use of other drugs that showed significant effects in Table 5. If such cases were removed from the analysis, the OR for vitamin B12 decreased to 1.14 (95% CI 0.76-1.70) and was thus no longer statistically significant (Table 6). Folic acid did not decrease the risk for a septum defect (Table 5). An explanation could be that folic acid was often given to patients using drugs which could increase the septum defect risk, e.g., anticonvulsants. When such women and women with diabetes were excluded from the analysis, the OR declined a little but was still not significantly low (Table 6).

Table 8. Effect of maternal use of antidepressants on the risk for a septum defect in the child according to type of drug. Number of children with septum defects = 7 308, total number of children in population = 1 282 858. Odds ratio (OR) with 95% confidence intervals (95% CI), adjusted for year of birth, maternal age, parity, smoking, and BMI. Bold Figures mark statistical significance (p<0.05)

Antidepressant Group	Antidepressant	No. of exposed infants with septum defects	No. of exposed infants in population	OR/RR	95%CI
TCA	All	14	1292	**1.95**	**1.16-3.27**
	Clomipramine	9	828	1.97	0.90-3.75[#]
SSRI	All	75	12292	1.05	0.83-1.32
	Fluoxetine	11	1951	0.97	0.53-1.76
	Citalopram	30	4442	1.18	0.82-1.69
	Paroxetine	14	1110	**2.15**	**1.18-3.61**[#]
	Sertraline	18	4225	0.73	0.46-1.16
SNRI/NRI	All	13	1810	1.23	0.71-2.12
	Venlafaxine	7	1131	1.10	0.44-2.26[#]

[#] Risk ratio (RR) as observed over expected number with exact 95% CI.; SNRI/NRI = serotonin-noradrenalin/noradrenalin reuptake inhibitors; SSRI = selective serotonin reuptake inhibitors; TCA = tricyclic antidepressants.

Antihypertensive Drugs

Table 7 summarizes data on the association between the use of antihypertensive drugs and septum defects. There seems to be a stronger effect on ASD (alone or with VSD) than on isolated VSD. Beta-blocking agents seem to have a weaker effect on ASD than other anti-hypertensives. Only one of the exposed children had another major congenital malformation (2.1

expected). This effect disappeared nearly completely when mothers with diabetes or concomitant use of other drugs which increased the risk for septum defects, were removed from the analysis (Table 6). The main effect was from maternal diabetes – if only diabetic mothers were removed, 25 children with septum defects and exposed to antihypertensive drugs remained. The resulting OR was 1.29 (95% CI 0.87-1.91). On the other hand, analysis of the effect of diabetes after removal of women who used antihypertension drugs remained high. OR = 3.18 (95% CI 2.48-4.08).

Ovulation Stimulation

There is a non-significantly increased risk for any septum defect after the use of ovarian stimulation. When analyzed according to septum type, the RR just reached statistical significance for VSD (RR = 1.87, 95% CI 1.00-3.20) while no effect was seen for ASD (RR = 0.70, 95% CI 0.09-2.82) but the two estimates overlap. The effect on any septum defect was similar after maternal use of clomiphene (RR = 1.36, 95% CI 0.89-2.68) and gonadotropins (RR = 1.56, 95% CI 0.67-3.67), both estimates based on only 8 exposed cases each.

Thyroid Hormones

The risk increase is statistically significant for ASD (OR = 1.48, 95% CI 1.01-2.16) and lower and not statistically significant for VSD (OR = 1.13, 95% CI 0.89-1.45) or VSD+ASD (OR = 1.21, 95% CI 0.75-2.02). Nine exposed infants had another major congenital malformation (8.2 expected). When women with diabetes or using concomitant drugs with an effect on septum defects were removed from the analysis, the risk estimate changed only little but the remaining OR was no longer statistically significant (Table 6).

Antibiotics

The effect on any septum defect is low and not statistically significant, but the lower confidence limit is 0.90. The ORs for VSD (1.13) and for ASD (1.06) do not differ significantly. The majority of exposures consist of penicillins (61%) where the OR for any septum defect is 1.00 (95% CI 0.81-1.23). Among the other classes of antibiotics, elevated OR/RRs (although not statistically significant) were found for tetracyclines (RR = 1.45, 95% CI 0.79-2.43), for macrolides (RR = 1.47, 95% CI 0.78-2.51), nitrofurantoine (OR = 1.26, 95% CI 0.86-1.87) and for cephalosporines (RR = 1.54, 95% CI 0.82-2.63). The dominating macrolide drug, erythromycin, had a RR = 1.59 (95% CI 0.85-2.71). Among the 13 septum defects after exposure to cephalosporines, 11 were VSD (RR = 1.89, 95% CI 0.94-3.38). Among 738 women reporting the use of trimethoprim (± sulfonamide) only one had a child with a septum defect (expected number 4.2).

Immunosuppressive Drugs

The rather strongly increased risk for any septum defect is high and statistically significant for ASD (RR = 6.33, 95% CI 2.06-14.8) and is increased but not statistically significant for VSD (RR = 2.28, 95% CI 0.84-4.97) or VSD+ASD (RR = 3.57, 95% CI 0.43-12.9). None of the exposed children had another major congenital malformation. The total risk increase was based on 13 infants with septum defects, 12 of which were exposed to azathioprine (RR = 3.89, 95% CI 2.01-6.81). Azathioprine represented 561 of the 719 exposed individuals in the population. The effect of immunosuppressive drugs declined after removal of women with diabetes or concomitant use of drugs with an effect on septum defects. The remaining OR was still high but not statistically significant (Table 6).

NSAID

There was no increased risk for a septum defect after use of any NSAID. The estimated OR was higher for VSD (OR = 1.20, 95% CI 0.95-1.50) than for ASD (OR = 0.70, 95% CI 0.39-1.17) but the two ORs obviously do not differ. As an effect has been discussed concerning ibuprofen, a separate analysis was made for that drug, but no significantly increased risk was seen (OR = 1.05, 95% CI 0.83-1.34), for VSD 1.24 (95% CI 0.95-1.63).

Anticonvulsants

The risk increase for VSD was not statistically significant (OR = 1.35, 95% CI 0.80-2.27) while the risk for ASD was (OR = 3.86, 95% CI 1.99-

6.74). Only two infants had both VSD and ASD (2.5 expected). For carbamazepine no increased risk for any septum defect was seen but the confidence interval was large (RR = 1.00, 95% CI 0.37-2.18) while for valproic acid a strong and statistically significant risk was found (RR = 3.87, 95% CI 2.06-6.62), especially marked for ASD (RR = 9.84, 95% CI 3.61-21.4, based on only 6 cases).

Among the 28 exposed cases, six had at least one more major congenital malformation. The expected number is 1.42 and the RR = 4.23, 95% CI 1.55-9.20). The remaining 22 cases that had no further major malformation showed an OR = 1.50 (95% CI 0.99-2.27).

The risk declined somewhat after removal of women with diabetes or concomitant use of other drugs with an effect on the septum risk. It was still elevated but statistical significance was not reached (Table 6).

Antidepressants

For antidepressants as a whole, no increased risk for any septum defect is seen. When the drugs are divided into three main groups, only tricyclic antidepressants which make up only a small part of antidepressants show a significant risk increase (Table 8). There is no difference in effect of tricyclic drugs between the different septum defect types and none of the estimated risk ratios reached statistical significance. For VSD the RR was 1.74 (95% CI 0.75-3.43), for ASD 2.30 (95% CI 0.63-5.89), and for VSD+ASD 2.11 (95% CI 0.25-7.60). All three estimates can obviously refer to the same common risk. Two thirds of the exposures were from clomipramine − the RR for this specific drug was close to that for all tricyclic drugs. Only few cases were removed when women with diabetes or concomitant use of drugs with an effect on septum risk were excluded from the analysis but the remaining RR did not quite reach statistical significance (Table 6).

For SSRI drugs, no increased risk for any septum defect was seen, neither for VSD, ASD or VSD+ASD even though the estimate for ASD was the highest one (OR = 1.42, 95% CI 0.93-2.16) (Table 8). When the four main SSRI drugs were analyzed separately, only one reached statistical significance, paroxetine. The highest risk estimate was for VSD+ASD followed by isolated ASD but these estimates were based on few cases and the difference between the groups could be random (exact p = 0.18). Exclusion from the analysis of women with diabetes or concomitant use of other drugs with an effect on septum defect risk reduced the exposed number of children only little and the RR actually increased a little and remained statistically significant.

Drugs for Rhinitis

No sign of an increased risk was seen in Table 5. In the literature, oral decongestants have been discussed as carrying a risk. The OR for such oral drugs was 0.88 (95% CI 0.52-1.49) and for nose drops 1.08 (95% CI 0.83-1.41).

Antiasthmatics

For the total group, only a slight risk increase was seen for any septum defect but the lower confidence limit was 0.96. When more specific groups of anti-asthmatics were analyzed, none showed a statistically significant risk. The risk estimate for adrenergic drugs was slightly higher (OR = 1.15, 95% CI 0.98-1.34) than for inhaled steroids (OR = 1.03, 95% CI 0.82-1.29) but this difference could well be random. The effect of any anti-asthmatic drug was slightly lower for ASD (OR = 0.94, 95% CI 0.67-1.34) than for VSD (OR = 1.16, 95% CI 0.97-1.39) or VSD+ASD (OR = 1.15, 95% CI 0.77-1.73) but these differences could obviously be random.

Antihistamines

There was no sign of a risk increase for this group. Some of these drugs are specifically used for nausea and vomiting in pregnancy (NVP) and other are used mainly for allergy. The drugs used for NVP had a non-significantly protective effect for any septum defect (OR = 0.92, 95% CI 0.81-1.06) while the drugs used for allergy showed no effect at all (OR = 1.00, 95% CI 0.80-1.25).

Miscellaneous Drugs

Some further drugs have been linked to the origin of cardiovascular defects. Cytotoxic drugs are possible teratogens. In the present study, only 84 women reported the use of this category of drugs – three of the children had septum defects, RR = 6.38 (95% CI 1.32-18.7). One of these women had use cyclophosphamide and the child had VSD+ASD. Two women had used mercaptopurine; one of the children had a VSD, the other an ASD.

Use of aspirin has been linked to cardiovascular defects [13]. In the present study, 1570 women reported the use of this drug – there were six children with septum defects: RR = 0.67 (95% CI 0.35-1.46). A combination of codeine and acetyl salicylic acid or paracetamol was reported by 1533 women. Ten of the children had septum defects (RR = 1.05, 95% CI 0.51-1.94).

The teratogenic effect of antifungal drugs and notably high doses of fluconazole has been discussed [14]. A total of 570 women reported the use of fluconazole in early pregnancy, three of the children had septum defects (RR = 1.05, 95% CI 0.51-1.94).

DISCUSSION

Problems with the Ascertainment of Cardiac Septum Defects

Septum defects are common malformations and therefore offer good possibilities for study. This is hampered by the fact that the diagnosis and recording may be inexact, notably of less severe forms. In the present study, the most uncertain source of information is probably the MBR, where the diagnosis is the result of a pediatric examination shortly after birth. If cases are recorded only in MBR it is likely that some of the recorded diagnoses were incorrect or represented VSD which closed spontaneously. This would mean that a number of non-malformed infants were included in the case series which will reduce the size of an OR estimate for a harmful factor. When cases which were only ascertained from MBR were removed from the analysis, the OR estimates increased only slightly, however.

On the other hand, some cases of VSD or ASD may have been missed – some of them may not give symptoms until later in life. This phenomenon will reduce the estimates of the prevalence of the malformations but will hardly affect risk estimates. Such infants will be allocated to the group of control infants but will make up a very small part of them.

A common problem when only infants are studied is the possibility that some defects have been detected prenatally and this has resulted in pregnancy interruption. This must be a rare situation for fetuses with only VSD or ASD but may be relevant for fetuses where the septum defect was combined with another major malformation which is detectable prenatally and may result in a pregnancy termination. Among the 888 infants (12%) with another diagnosis than VSD and/or ASD, serious malformations which could result in prenatal detection followed by abortion occurred in 63, less than 1%. How many exposed fetuses that were actually aborted and therefore missed in the study is not known.

Advantages with the Present Study Design

An advantage with the present study is its large size and that the information on maternal characteristics and drug use was obtained by interviews in early pregnancy, before anyone knew about the presence of a congenital malformation. The information was thus obtained prospectively related to the knowledge of the septum defects and recall or interviewer bias were therefore avoided. A draw-back is that generally no prior hypothesis existed and a large number of comparisons were made which can give false statistical significances as a result of multiple testing.

Maternal Characteristics and Cardiac Septum Defects

Among maternal characteristics which affected the risk for a cardiac septum defect high maternal age ($\geq$ 35 years) and first parity had weak but statistically significant effects, similar for VSD and ASD. The effect of maternal smoking was marked only for ASD while the effect of maternal overweight or obesity were especially related to VSD. An increased risk in women who had reported a period of unwanted childlessness (notably 3 years or more) was seen at ASD.

Characterization of Children with Cardiac Septum Defects

Children with septum defects were more often than expected born preterm, were female, and were born in multiple births. None of these characteristics acts as a confounder as no effect on drug use can exist. Multiple births could be a mediating factor for drugs which affect the probability for twinning, e.g., ovarian stimulation.

Nearly 9% of all children with septum defects also had another congenital malformation. For most of the analyzed drugs which showed an excess risk of a septum defect, only few exposed children had another major malformation and it is not possible from this material to see if there is a difference in effect on isolated septum defects and on septum defects associated with other major malformations. The only indicated difference is for children exposed to anticonvulsants when 27% also had other congenital malformations. The risk increase after anticonvulsants seemed larger for the group with other major congenital malformations than for the group of isolated septum defects and the latter was not quite statistically significant. The association between maternal use of anticonvulsants and an increased risk for septum defects therefore seems to be related to the general teratogenic effect of these drugs, especially strong for valproic acid. It is also possible that the detection and registration of mild septum defects was increased when the child had other malformations.

Concomitantly Used Drugs

Maternal drug use of a drug can be associated with septum defects through an effect from concomitantly used drugs. If drug A is used together with drug B more often than expected and drug B has an effect of its own on the septum defect risk, this can result in a non-causal association between drug A and septum defects. An example could have been the use of anticonvulsants as mood stabilizers together with antidepressants.

In an effort to eliminate this, analyses were made excluding women with diabetes or with concomitant use of any other drug which in itself was associated with an increased risk of a septum defect. This will at the same time reduce the number of exposed cases and therefore the power of the study and will result in widened confidence intervals. As seen in Table 6, most risk estimates were reduced by this manipulation. Some of them remained high but lost statistical significance. It is then not possible to draw the conclusion that the crude effect was completely due to this type of confounding. It is still possible that the original estimate is correct and that the loss of statistical significance was only an effect of the reduction of the size of the material.

This phenomenon seems to be the major reason for the observed association between vitamin B12 and septum defects – when women with diabetes or concomitant use of drugs with an effect on the risk for septum defects were removed from the analysis, the association with vitamin B12 use declined markedly and was no longer statistically significant. It seems rather unlikely that this vitamin could have a harmful effect of its own.

The use of folic acid was not associated with a decreased risk for a septum defect. When the analyses was repeated after removal of women with diabetes or concomitant use of drugs with an effect on septum risk, the OR declined somewhat but was still not statistically significant (Table 6).

Confounding by Indication

Another reason for an observed drug effect could be confounding by indication [15]. This may be true for antihypertensive drugs where the effect seemed to be mainly associated with maternal diabetes which was present in nearly half of the exposed cases. It should be pointed out that women with diabetes were removed from the analysis in the study by Lennestål et al. [7] where an effect of antihypertensives was demonstrated on the risk of a cardiovascular defect (but septum defects were not specifically studied).

Antihypertensive drug use has repeatedly been associated with an increased risk for cardivacular defects including septum defects [4]. One paper [16] described an effect of antihypertensive drugs belonging to the ACE inhibitor type compared with other antihypertensive drugs. Another study [7] found similar effects on the cardiac defect risk for ACE inhibitors and beta-blockers, when used as antihypertensives. In the present study, the effect was much lower for beta-blockers than for ACE inhibitors and angiotensin II blockers. Beta-blockers, however, are not only used at hypertension but also at other conditions (like migraine) and then often at lower dosage which can contribute to the lower effect. Caton et al. [4] compared women with treated or untreated hypertension and found a difference in teratogenic effect, but the severity of the underlying disease probably differs between these two groups.

A typical example when the observed association most likely is due to the underlying pathology is thyroxin. It seems unlikely that this hormone, which is used as substitution at hypothyroidism, can cause a malformation. It is more likely that the increased hormone demand in early pregnancy can result in hypothyroidism which may affect development. This possibility is discussed by Norstedt Wikner et al. [17]. In this paper, an OR for VSD or ASD after thyroxin exposure was 1.25 (not quite statistically significant), in the present study 1.22 but statistically significant. Removal of women with diabetes or concomitant use of other drugs with an effect on the septum risk changed the OR only moderately but statistical significance was lost (lower confidence limit 0.96). Another paper which suggested an association was that by Robert et al. [18].

The not quite statistically significant risk increase after ovulation stimulation may in a similar way be confounded by an increased risk of septum defects among children born of women who reported a period of unwanted childlessness. The complex relationship between subfertility, ovarian stimulation, and in vitro fertilization (where also an increased risk for septum defects has been described [19]) makes it difficult to disentangle causality but much data argue in favor of the idea that the increased risk for a congenital malformation is mainly associated with parental subfertility [20].

A confounding by indication is also a possible explanation of the effects of aminosalicylic drugs and immunosuppressive drugs as was discussed by Cleary and Källén [21] who also found a three times increased risk for VSD and/or ASD after maternal use of azathioprine, based on partially the same material as that used in the present study (years 1995-2007 in the Cleary and Källén study and 1998-2010 in the present study). A direct teratogenic effect notably of azathioprine is also possible.

Direct Drug Effects?

A confounding by indication is less likely to explain the apparently specific effects of two antidepressants: clomipramine and paroxetine. Even though the indications of usage may differ somewhat between these drugs and other antidepressants, the marked differences in risks speak in favor of drug effects. Clomipramine can inhibit a specific cardiac potassium (IKr) channel, expressed by a hERG related gene [22], which may explain an effect of embryonic cardiac arrhythmia, resulting in pressure changes and misdirection of blood flow and some cardiovascular defects [23].

The possible effect of paroxetine has been much discussed since the first signals appeared [24, 25]. Previous studies of the Swedish data indicated a specific effect of paroxetine on cardiovascular defects and cardiac septum defects which was significantly stronger than the non-significant effects seen with other SSRI drugs [10, 26]. Some other studies have reached a similar conclusion (e.g., [27]) while other studies either found a general harmful effect of all SSRIs [9, 28] or no effect at all [29]. Two studies [30, 31] suggested an association between maternal use of fluoxetine and cardiovascular defects. The variable results in different studies may be explained by methodological problems, e.g., by the fact that infants born of women who have used antidepressants during pregnancy have a higher risk to get neonatal inpatient care than other infants due to neonatal mortality. If data are basically obtained from neonatal discharge diagnoses [9, 28], this may bias the results.

The increased risk for septum defects among children born of women using cytostatic drugs is also probably a direct effect, but only few women reported the use of such drugs.

Anticonvulsant drugs are well-known teratogens, best known for valproic acid. The teratogenic effect of valproic acid is relatively broad with an increased risk of, for instance, spina bifida, cardiovascular defects, and hypospadias. In the present study, the effect on septum defects was clear and was strongest for valproic acid when other major malformations existed. It is likely that the teratogenic effect seen after the use of anticonvulsants is caused by the drugs and is not confounded by indication. Removal from the analysis of women with diabetes or with concomitant use of other drugs with an effect on septum defect risk reduced the number of exposed children only little (Table 6), the OR remained elevated but not quite statistically significant (lower confidence limit 0.96).

Another problem where data in the literature vary concerns NSAIDs. In retrospective case-control studies, use of NSAID and notably ibuprofen was associated with an increased risk of septum defects [3]. Ericson and Källén [32] found an increased risk of cardiovascular defects among infants born of women who used NSAID in early pregnancy and a majority of these defects were septum defects. There was no drug specificity. In the present study, this finding was not verified. Either the first observation was random in spite of formal statistical significance (as a result of multiple testing) or the explanation may lie in a change in NSAID usage. In Sweden these drugs became over-the-counter drugs and were recommended for temporary pain or similar indications. As long as they were prescription drugs, usage was much less frequent and perhaps underlying conditions (e.g., rheumatic disease or other chronic illness) may have resulted in the use of higher dosage and more extended treatment periods than what is the case more recently.

Antibiotics and Common Infections

There was no evidence that use of common antibiotic drugs could increase the risk for septum defects. Some risk estimates were elevated but none reached statistical significance. A study suggested an increased risk of septum defects after maternal use of erythromycin [33] – the estimated OR was 1.69

(95% CI 1.06-2.69) which is rather similar to the present estimate: 1.59. The two studies overlap during the period 1998-2002, that is four among the 13 years of the present study. The tentative explanation to this association was similar to that mentioned for clomipramine (see above), an inhibition of a specific cardiac potassium (IKr) channel.

There was no sign of a harmful effect of trimethoprim in spite of its alleged effect on folic acid metabolism but only 738 women had used this drug and the expected number of septum defects was only four. It has repeatedly been stated in the literature that maternal febrile illness could increase the risk for cardiovascular defects including VSD [6] but these conclusions were based on retrospective studies. If true, one would expect an effect of use of penicillins which are often prescribed for upper respiratory infections, but no such effect was seen in the present material.

CONCLUSION

To conclude, some maternal characteristics are associated with an increased risk for offspring cardiac septum defects. These include some chronic diseases and notably maternal diabetes. In addition there is some evidence that a direct teratogenic effect is seen of a few drugs, e.g., anticonvulsants, clomipramine, paroxetine, and cytostatics. The distinction between the effect of the drug and of the underlying disease is often difficult to make.

REFERENCES

[1]   Tikkanen J., Heinonen O. P. Risk factors for ventricular septal defects in Finland. *Public Health* 1991; 105: 99-112.

[2]   Tikkanen J., Heinonen O. P. Risk factors for atrial septal defects. *Eur J Epidemiol* 1992; 8: 509-515.

[3]   Ferencz C., Loffredo C. A., Correa-Villaseñor A., Wilson P. D. Genetic and Environmental Risk Factors of Major Cardiovascular Malformations. The Baltimore-Washington Infant Study 1981-1989. *Persp Ped Cardiol* 1997; 5: 1-463.

[4]   Caton A. R., Bell E. M., Druschel C. M., Werler M. M., Lin A. E., Browne M. L., McNutt L-A., Romitti P. A. Mitchell A. A., Olney R. S.,

Correa A. Antihyprtensive medication use duriing pregnancy and the risk of cardiovascular malformations. *Hypertension* 2009; 54: 63-70.

[5] Källén B., Otterblad Olausson P. Maternal drug use in early pregnancy and infant cardiovascular defect. *Reprod Toxicol* 2003; 17: 255-261.

[6] Jenkins K. J., Correa A., Feinstein J. A., Botto L., Britt A. E., Daniels S. R., Elixson M., Warnes C. A., Webb C. L. Noninherited risk factors and congenital cardiovascular defects: Current knowledge. *Circulation* 2007; 115: 2995-3014.

[7] Lennestål R., Otterblad Olausson P., Källén B. Maternal use of antihypertensive drugs in early pregnancy and delivery outcome, notably the presence of congenital heart defects in the infants. *Eur J Clin Pharmacol* 2009; 65: 615-625.

[8] Pedersen L. H., Henriksen T. B., Vestergaard M., Olsen J., Bech B. H. Selective serotonin reuptake inhibitors in pregnancy and congenital malformations: population based cohort study, *BMJ* 2009; 339: b3569. Doi: 10.1136/bmjb3569.

[9] Kornum J. B., Nielsen R. B., Pedersen L., Mortensen P. B., Nørgaard M. Use of selective serotonin-reuptake inhibitors during early pregnancy and risk of congenital malformations: updated analysis. *Clin Epidemiol* 2010; 2: 29.36.

[10] Reis M., Källén B. Delivery outcome after maternal use of antidepressant drugs in pregnancy: an update using Swedish data. *Psychol Med* 2010; 10: 1923-1733.

[11] National Board of Health and Welfare. Centre for Epidemiology. *Registration of congenital malformations in Swedish health registers.* 2004. (http://www.socialstyrel-sen.se/Publikationer2004/ 2004-112-1). Accessed September 12, 2012.

[12] National Board of Health and Welfare. Centre for Epidemiology. *The Swedish Medical Birth Register – A summary of content and quality.* 2003. (http://www.socialstyrelsen. se/Publikationer 2003/2003-112-3) Accessed September 12, 2012.

[13] Aleck K. A., Bartley D. L. Multiple malformation syndrome following fluconazole use in pregnancy; report of an additional patient. *Am J Med Genet* 1997; 72: 253-256.

[14] Werler M. M., Mitchell A. A., Shapiro S. The relation of aspirin use during the first trimester of pregnancy to congenital cardiac defects. *N Engl J Med* 1989; 321: 137-147.

[15] Källén B. The problem of confounding in studies of the effect of maternal drug use on pregnancy outcome. *Obst Gynecol Internat* 2012; doi.10.1155/2012/148616.

[16] Cooper W. O., Hernandez-Diaz S., Arbogast P. et al. Major congenital malformations after first- trimester exposure to ACE inhibitors. *N Engl J Med* 2006; 354: 2443-2451.

[17] Norstedt Wikner B., Skjöldebrand Sparre L., Stiller C-O., Källén B., Asker C. Maternal use of thyroid hormones and neonatal outcome. *Acta Obstet Gynecol* 2008; 87: 617-627.

[18] Robert E., Vollset S. E., Botto L., Lancaster P. A. J., Merlob P., Mastroiacovo P., Cocchi G., Ashisawa M., Sakamoto S., Orioli I. Malformation surveillance and mater-nal drug exposure: the MADRE project. *Int J Risk Safety Med* 1994; 6: 75-118.

[19] Källén B., Finnström O., Nygren K. G., Otterblad Olausson P. In vitro fertilization (IVF) in Sweden: risk for congenital malformations after different IVF methods. *Birth Def Res* (Part A) 2005; 73: 162-169.

[20] Rimm A. A., Katayama A. C., Katayama K. P. A meta-analysis of the impact of IVF and ICSI on major malformations after adjusting for the effect of subfertility. *J Assist Reprod Genet* 2011; 28: 699-705.

[21] Cleary B. J., Källén B. Early pregnancy azathioprine use and pregnancy outcome. *Birth Def Res* (Part A) 2009; 85: 647-654.

[22] Jo S. H., Hong H. K., Chong S. H., Won K. H., Jung S. J., Choe H. Clomipramine block of the hERG K+ channel: accessibility to F656 and Y652. *Eur J Pharmacol* 2008; 592: 19-25.

[23] Danielsson B. R., Sköld A., Azarbayjani F. Class III antiarrhythmics and phenytoin teratogenicity due to embryonic cardiac dysrhythmia and reoxygenation damage, *Curr Pharm Des* 2001; 7: 787-802.

[24] *GSK:* See http://ctr.gsk.cp.uk/Summary/paroxetine/studylist.asp.

[25] Diav-Citrin O., Shechtman S., Weinbaum D., Arnon J., di Giantonio E., Clementi M., Ornoy A.. Paroxetine and fluoxetine in pregnancy: a multicentre prospective, controlled study, *Reprod Toxicol* 2005; 20: 459 (Abstract).

[26] Källén B., Otterblad Olausson P. Maternal use of selective serotonin re-uptake inhibitors in early pregnancy and infant congenital malformations. *Birth Def Res* (Part A) 2007; 79: 301-308.

[27] Bérard A., Ramos É., Rey E., Blais L., St.-André M., Oraichi D. First trimester exposure to paroxetine and risk of cardiac malformations in infants; the importance of dosage. *Birth Def Res* (Part B) 2007, 80. 18-27.

[28] Jimenez-Solem E., Andersen J. T., Petersen M., Broedbaek K., Krogh Jensen J., Afzal S., Gislason G. H., Torp-Pedersen C., Poulsen H. E. Exposure to selective serotonin reuptake inhibitors and the risk of congenital malformations: a nationwide cohort study. *BMJ Open* 2012: 2e00148. Doi: 10.1136/ bmjopen-2012-001148.

[29] Oberlander T., Warburton W., Misri S., Riggs W., Aghajanian J., Hertzman C. Major congenital malformations following prenatal exposure to serotonin reuptake inhibitors and benzodiazepines using population-based health data. *Birth Defects Res* (Part B) 2008; 83:68-76.

[30] Malm H., Klaukka T., Neuvonen P. J. Risks associated with selective serotonin reuptake inhibitors in pregnancy. *Obstet Gynecol* 2005; 106: 1289-1296.

[31] Diav-Citrin O., Shechtman S., Weinbaum D., Wajnberg R., Avgil M., di Gianantonio E., Clementi M., Weber-Schoendorfer C., Schaefer C., Ornoy A. Paroxetine and fluoxetine in pregnancy: a prospective, multicentre, controlled, observational study. *Brit J Clin Pharmacol* 2008; 65: 695-705.

[32] Ericson A., Källén B. Nonsteroidal anti-inflammatory drugs in early pregnancy, *Reprod Toxicol* 2001; 15: 371-375.

[33] Källén B., Otterblad Olausson P., Danielsson B. R. Is erythromycin therapy teratogenic in humans? *Reprod Toxicol* 2005; 20: 209-214.

In: Atrial and Ventricular Septal Defects
Editor: Steven A. Larkin

ISBN: 978-1-62618-326-1
© 2013 Nova Science Publishers, Inc.

Chapter 3

NON-SURGICAL CLOSURE OF ATRIAL SEPTAL DEFECTS IN CHILDREN

P. Syamasundar Rao[*]

Professor of Pediatrics and Medicine
Director, Pediatric Cardiology Fellowship Programs
Emeritus Chief of Pediatric Cardiology,
University of Texas-Houston Medical School
Houston, TX, US

ABSTRACT

There are four types of *atrial septal* defects (ASDs) namely, ostium secundum, ostium primum, sinus venosus and coronary sinus ASDs. Patent foramen ovale (PFO) is present in nearly one third of normal population, thus making the PFO a normal variant, although it may become important in certain situations and will not be the subject of this review. In this review management of only ostium secundum ASDs is discussed. Whereas surgical intervention was used in the past, transcatheter methods are currently used for closure of ostium secundum ASDs. A large number of devices have been developed over the last three and one-half decades. Some of the devices have been discontinued and

[*] Address for correspondence: Dr. P. Syamasundar Rao, Professor and Emeritus Chief of Pediatric Cardiology, The University of Texas/Houston Medical School, 6410 Fannin, UTPB Suite 425, Houston, TX 77030, USA; Phone: 713-500-5738; Fax: 713-500-5751, E-mail: P.Syamasundar.Rao@uth.tmc.edu.

others modified and redesigned. Clinical trials have been undertaken with a large number of devices and feasibility, safety and effectiveness of these devices in occluding the ASD have been demonstrated. At the present time however, Amplatzer Septal Occluder, Amplatzer Cribriform Device and HELEX devices are the only devices that are approved for general clinical use by the FDA. The experience with Amplatzer for most defects has been encouraging. HELEX device is only useful in small to medium-sized defects. Historical aspects of device development, indications for intervention, the method of device implantation, immediate and follow-up results (along with complications), including our own personal experience with Amplatzer device in over 150 patients and a comparison with surgery will be presented. It may be concluded that Amplatzer device may be the best available option at the present time. Careful attention to the details of the technique is mandatory to achieve a successful outcome.

Keywords: Atrial septal defect, non-surgical closure, Amplatzer septal occluder, HELEX Device, Amplatzer cribriform device

INTRODUCTION

Atrial septal defects (ASDs) cause left to right shunt because the left atrial pressure is higher than that in the right atrium. This results in volume overloading of the right ventricle. This is generally well tolerated in infancy and childhood but, development of exercise intolerance and arrhythmias in later childhood and adolescence, and the risk for development of pulmonary vascular obstructive disease in adulthood make ASDs important. Four major types of ASDs are described and include ostium secundum, ostium primum, sinus venosus and coronary sinus defects. In this review I will address non-surgical, transcatheter occlusion of ostium secundum ASDs.

Persistent patency of the foramen ovale in nearly one third of normal population makes the patent foramen ovale (PFO) a normal variant. However, the PFOs become important in the presence of other structural abnormalities of the heart or when they become the seat of right to left shunt causing paradoxical embolism resulting in stroke/transient ischemic attacks or other problems, such as migraine, Caisson's disease and platypnea-orthodexia syndrome. The issues related to PFOs will not be reviewed in this chapter.

Atrial septal defects constitute 8% to 13% of all congenital heart defects (CHDs). There is deficiency of the septal tissue in the region of fossa ovalis. These defects may be small, medium or large. Single defects are usual, although, occasionally multiple defects and fenestrated defects can also be present. Because of left-to-right shunting across the defect, the right heart structures are dilated and somewhat hypertrophied. Pulmonary vascular obstructive changes are not usually seen until adulthood.

ASD patients are usually asymptomatic and are most often detected at the time of preschool physical. On examination the right ventricular and right ventricular outflow tract impulses are increased and hyperdynamic. The second heart sound is widely split and fixed (splitting does not vary with respiration) and is the most characteristic sign of ASD. An ejection systolic murmur of grade I-II/VI intensity is heard best at the left upper sternal border. A grade I-II/VI mid-diastolic flow rumble is heard with the bell of the stethoscope at the left lower sternal border; this is secondary to large volume flow across the tricuspid valve. Chest X-ray with mild to moderate cardiomegaly, prominent main pulmonary artery segment and increased pulmonary vascular markings and electrocardiogram with mild right ventricular hypertrophy with rsR' pattern in the right chest leads is suggestive of the diagnosis. Echocardiogram showing dilatation of the right ventricle, two dimensional demonstration of the defect in the atrial septum and color Doppler imaging with left to right shunt (Figure 1) confirms the diagnosis.

The management of ASD in children is largely dependent of the age at presentation, presence of congestive heart failure and the size of the defect. Congestive heart failure is rare with ASDs, but when present, these infants should receive anti-congestive measures (diuretics and digoxin). If they do not improve, surgical and more recently trans-catheter intervention to close the defects is considered. Surgical closure of ostium secundum ASDs is safe and effective with low (<1%) mortality. However, the morbidity associated with sternotomy/thoracotomy, cardiopulmonary bypass and potential for postoperative complications cannot be avoided. Other disadvantages of surgical therapy are the expense associated with surgical correction, residual surgical scar and psychological trauma to the patients and/or the parents. Because of these reasons several trans-catheter methods have been developed [1,2]. In the current era, surgical repair is largely reserved for defects with poor septal rims in which the interventional cardiologist deems that defect is difficult to close with trans-catheter methodology or was unsuccessful in closing the defect. In addition, if intra-cardiac repair of other defects is contemplated, surgical closure of ASD should be performed at the same time.

In this review non-surgical, transcatheter closure of *ASDs* in children is discussed.

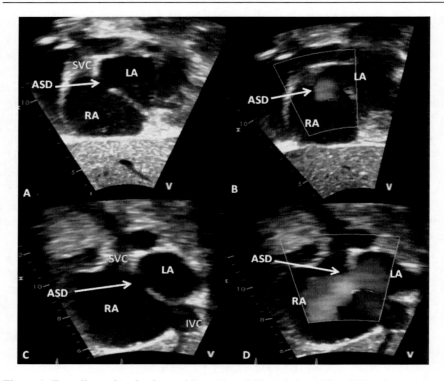

Figure 1. Two dimensional subcostal long (A and B) and short (C and D) axis trans-thoracic echocardiographic views of the atrial septum demonstrating secundum atrial septal defect (ASD) in the atrial septum (left panels) and color Doppler with left to right shunt (right panels). IVC, inferior vena cava; LA, left atrium; RA, right atrium; SVC, superior vena cava.

INDICATIONS FOR TRANSCATHTER OOCLUSION

Even though there may not be any symptoms at presentation, occlusion of moderate to large ASDs is generally recommended so as to: 1) prevent development of pulmonary vascular obstructive disease later in adulthood, 2) reduce probability for development of supra-ventricular arrhythmias and 3) avoid development of symptoms during adolescence and adulthood. Elective closure around age 4 to 5 years is suggested. ASD closure during infancy is not undertaken unless the infant is symptomatic. Right ventricular volume overloading by echocardiogram and a Qp:Qs >1.5 (if the child had cardiac catheterization) are indications for closure.

HISTORICAL ASPECTS

The first three devices used to close ASDs will be detailed followed by a listing of the subsequently developed devices.

King's Device

King and Mills [3] described a device composed of paired, Dacron-covered stainless steel umbrellas collapsed into a capsule at the tip of a catheter and used it to occlude ASDs that were created by a punch biopsy technique in adult dogs. Endothelialization of the implanted umbrellas was observed during the follow-up. The technique was then extended to human subjects [4,5].

Rashkind's Devices

Rashkind [6,7] developed a slightly different type of ASD closure device; the initial Rashkind umbrella consisted of three stainless-steel arms covered with foam which was later modified such that there are six stainless steel arms with the alternate arms carrying a miniature "fish" hook. An intricate centering mechanism, consisting of five arms bent to produce a gentle outward curve was incorporated into the device delivery system. The delivery mechanism is built on a 6 F catheter with locking tip, which interlocks with the central hub of the device. Excellent endothelialization of the umbrella components was demonstrated in animal models. Studies in human subjects followed [7,8]. Rashkind modified this device into double-disc prosthesis [8] because he identified problems with the hooked device; this modification was patterned after a patent ductus arteriosus occluding device [9] that he has concurrently developed. Lock and his associates [10] modified the device by introducing a second spring in center of the arms because of the inability of the umbrellas to fold back against each other; this modified device was named clamshell occluder. Following successful implantation in lambs, the procedure was extended to human subjects [11]. Clinical trials by these and other investigators continued but because of fractures of the arms of the device in 40 to 84% of devices with occasional embolization [12,13], further clinical trials with the device were suspended in 1991 by the FDA and the investigators.

Buttoned Devices

Sideris et al described "buttoned device" [14,15] at about the time of transformation of Rashkind double disk device to clamshell device. The device consisted of two components: occluder and counter-occluder. The occluder consisted of an x-shaped, Teflon-coated wire skeleton covered with 1/8-in polyurethane foam. The wire skeleton of the occluder can be folded, making the wires parallel, which can then be introduced into an 8-French sheath. When delivered to site of implantation, the occluder springs opens into its original square-shaped structure. A 2-mm string loop made of silk thread is attached to the center of the occluder; the loop is closed with a 1-mm knot (button). The counter-occluder is composed of a single strand, Teflon-coated wire skeleton covered with rhomboid shaped polyurethane foam. A rubber piece is sutured in its center and becomes a buttonhole. The device was manufactured in 5-mm increments beginning with 25-mm size. The device size was measured by the diagonal length of the occluder and is same as the length of the counter-occluder. This may be considered *first generation buttoned device*. Studies in piglets demonstrated full occlusion of the ASD and endothelialization of the device [14]. Based on preliminary clinical experience with this device [16], the device was modified by strengthening the button-loop by replacing the silk tie with 4-lb proof nylon and introducing a radio-opaque marker on the button (*second generation buttoned device*). The device was further modified by converting eccentric button to be aligned straight (*third-generation device*) and by introduction of an 8-mm string loop, attached to the occluder with two buttons (*fourth generation device*) [17,18], thus making it easier to button the occluder and counter-occluder across the atrial septum; this was patterned after the buttoned device for patent ductus arteriosus [19]. Concomitantly, a number of other modifications of the device were introduced which include, centering device [20] to center the device over the defect, inverted device [21] to address closure of right to left shunts, centering on demand device [22,23] to center the device when necessary and hybrid device [24] to address closure of defects with associated with atrial septal aneurysm. The device has also been successfully used to close atrial defects presumed to be responsible for paradoxical embolism and cerebrovascular accidents [25], patent foramen ovale causing hypoxemia in platypnea-orthodeoxia syndrome in the elderly [26] and persistent right to left shunt associated with previously operated complex congenital cardiac anomalies, including Fontan fenestrations [21]. A number of single institutional and multi-institutional clinical trials were undertaken which demonstrated feasibility, safety and effectiveness of this device [24]. However, pre-market-approval (PMA) application was not made and consequently the device is not approved by the FDA and is not available for general clinical use [27].

Subsequently Described Devices

Later a number of other devices were described [27] and these include, ASDOS (atrial septal defect occluding system), monodisk device, Das Angel Wing Device, Amplatzer septal occluder, CardioSEAL device, STARFlex device, Sideris' Wire-less devices including transcatheter patch, HELEX septal occluder, fenestrated Amplatzer device to keep atrial septal defects open to maintain cardiac output, cribriform device to occlude multiple or fenestrated ASDs, BioSTAR, nanoplatinum coating to prevents nickel release from Amplatzer devices, thus averting Kounis syndrome, Solysafe Septal Occluder device, BioTREK, Occlutech, ATRIASEPT I-ASD device, ATRIASEPT II-ASD and ULTRASEPT, The pfm ASD-R devices and others [27]. Other devices such as Cardi-O-Fix Septal Occluder, Heart R Septal Occluder, cocoon, Lifetech Scientific device (also called sears device), some manufactured in China and others that may have escaped detection by our literature search and may be in development [27].

Despite extensive studies with many of these devices, Amplatzer Septal Occluder and HELEX are the only two devices that are approved for general clinical use by the FDA. Amplatzer cribriform device to occlude multiple or fenestrated ASDs is also approved by the FDA. A number of other devices are in clinical trials either in the US or in other countries. The interested reader referred elsewhere [27,28] for a more detailed discussion of historical aspects of ASD closure devices.

Approved Devices (Figure 2)

As mentioned in the preceding section, only Amplatzer Septal Occluder and HELEX are approved by the FDA; these devices will be briefly described. Amplatzer cribriform device, a variant of Amplatzer Septal Occluder is also approved for closure fenestrated ASDs.

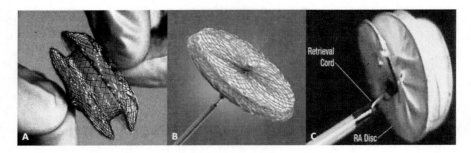

Figure 2. Photographs of the FDA approved devices: A. Amplatzer Septal Occluder, B. Amplatzer multi-fenestrated septal occluder (Cribriform device) and C. HELEX device. See text for detailed description of these devices.

Amplatzer Septal Occluder

Amplatzer Septal Occluder is a double disk device build with 0.004" to 0.007" Nitinol (nickle-titanium compound) wire with shape memory [29]. A 4 mm wide waist connects the left and right atrial disks for stenting the ASD. The left atrial disk is larger than the right (Figure 2A). Dacron polyester patches are sewn into each disk. Many sizes are available from the manufacturer (AGA); the device size is measured as the size of waist of the device.

They are available in 4 mm thru' 38 mm sizes; the 4 mm to 20 mm devices in one mm increments and 20 mm to 38 mm in two mm increments. The device can easily be withdrawn into a delivery sheath and can be implanted across the defect and if necessary pulled back into the sheath and repositioned.

Amplatzer Multi-Fenestrated Septal Occluder (Cribriform Device)

Amplatzer cribriform device (Figure 2B) is constructed similar to Amplatzer Septal Occluder and consists of equal-sized left and right discs connected with a thin waist [30,31]. Currently available sizes in the US are 18, 25, 30 and 35 mm; the device size is measured as the size of disc diameter of the device.

HELEX Device

HELEX device (Figure 2C) is made up of a single stand super-elastic, Nitinol wire frame with ultrathin poly-tetra-fluro-ethelene (ePTFE) covering the wire [32]. The delivery system has three components, a delivery catheter, control catheter and a mandrel. When deployed, it forms two interconnected round disks, intended to be placed on either side of the atrial septum. The device is available in 15 thru' 35 mm diameter sizes in 5 mm increments.

TECHNIQUE OF DEVICE IMPLANTATION

Initially percutaneous right heart catheterization is performed to confirm the clinical and echocardiographic diagnosis with particular attention to exclude partial anomalous pulmonary venous return. A left atrial cineangiogram in a left axial oblique view (30^0 LAO and 30^0 Cranial) with the catheter positioned in the right upper pulmonary vein at its junction with the left atrium is then carried out (Figure 3).

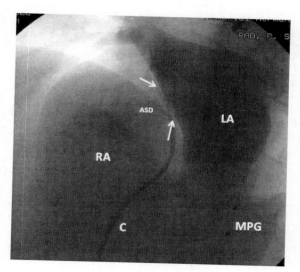

Figure 3. Selected cine frame from left atrial (LA) cineangiogram with the catheter (C) tip positioned at the LA/right pulmonary vein junction in a left axial oblique view (30^0 left anterior oblique and 30^0 cranial) demonstrating the atrial septal defect (ASD). The margins of the ASD are marked with arrows. MPG, marker pigtail catheter; RA, right atrium.

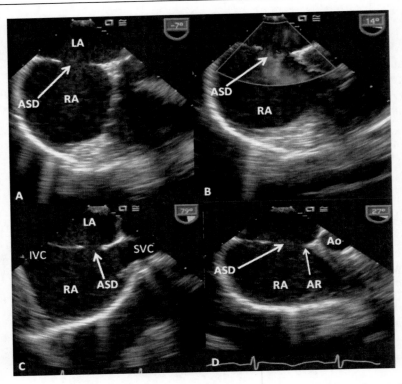

Figure 4. Selected two-dimensional (A, C and D) and color flow (B) video frames from a transesophageal echocardiographic (TEE) study of the atrial septum showing an atrial septal defect (ASD) in long axis (A) bi-caval (C) and short axis (D) views with left to right shunt (B). Note very small aortic (anterio-superior) rim (AR) in D. Ao, aorta; IVC, inferior vena cava; LA, left atrium; RA, right atrium; SVC, superior vena cava.

Then transesophageal (TEE) or intracardiac (ICE) echocardiography is performed to measure the size (Figures 4) and number (Figures 5 and 6) of the ASDs, to visualize entry of all pulmonary veins into the left atrium and to examine the atrial septal rims.

Whether TEE or ICE is used to measure the size of the defect and monitor the device placement is institutional and cardiologist dependent and both methods have advantages and disadvantages. The author of this chapter, however, prefers TEE. Static balloon sizing of the ASD using NuMed PTS or AGA Amplatzer sizing balloons is performed routinely by some cardiologists.

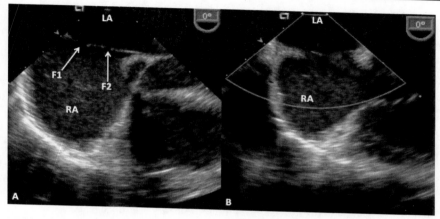

Figure 5. Selected two-dimensional (A) and color flow (B) video frames from a transesophageal echocardiographic (TEE) study of the atrial septum showing a fenestrated (F1 and F2) atrial septal defect (A) with left to right shunt (B). LA, left atrium; RA, right atrium.

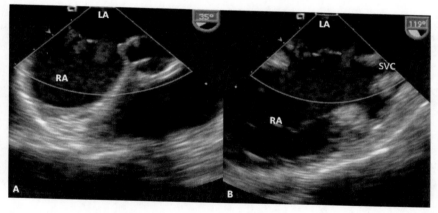

Figure 6. Selected color flow video frames from a transesophageal echocardiographic study in the same patient shown in figure 5 demonstrating three fenestrations in different echocardiographic views. LA, left atrium; RA, right atrium; SVC, superior vena cava.

However, we do not routinely perform balloon sizing, but rely on the echo sizing; we utilize the thick margins of the defect to measure the size of the ASD (Figure 7), leaving out the flail margins, a method similar to that suggested by Carcagnì and Presbitero [33].

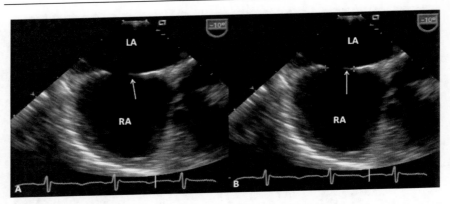

Figure 7. Selected two-dimensional video frames from a transesophageal echocardiographic study of the atrial septum showing thin margin (arrow) of the atrial septal defect (A) which is not included (B) in the measurement of the size of the defect. See text for details. LA, left atrium; RA, right atrium.

Systemic pressures are monitored throughout the procedure via an arterial line. Administration of heparin (100 units/kg) and monitoring the ACT to keep it above 200 seconds and of Ancef or a similar antibiotic are routine parts of the procedure. Aspirin 2 to 5 mg/kg as a single daily dose for six months is recommended in children. Clopidogrel (Plavix) may be used in adult patients.

Amplatzer Septal Occluder

An Amplatzer Septal Occluder 1 to 2 mm larger than the diameter of the ASD is selected for implantation. The size of delivery sheath accommodating the selected device is positioned in the left upper pulmonary vein, taking appropriate precautions to avoid inadvertent air entry into the system. The selected device is screwed onto the delivery cable; the device is loosened by unscrewing by one turn and drawn into the loader sheath under saline. The device is deposited into the delivery sheath while flushing the loader sheath continuously with a flushing solution. This is to prevent inadvertent air entry into the system. The device is advanced within the sheath under fluoroscopic guidance until it reaches the tip of the delivery sheath in the left upper pulmonary vein. The entire system is withdrawn until the tip of the sheath slips into the free left atrium and the device advanced, thus releasing the left atrial disk (Figures 8A and 9A).

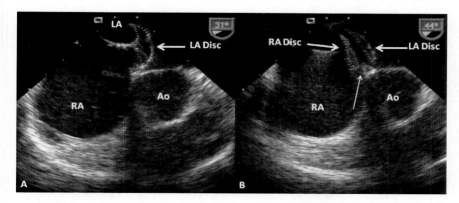

Figure 8. Selected two-dimensional video frames from a transesophageal echocardiographic study during the delivery of Amplatzer Septal Occluder with the left atrial disc (LA Disc) delivered (A) into left atrium (LA) and both the discs delivered (B) across the atrial septum. Note the aortic rim (thin arrow) is sandwiched between LA and right atrial (RA) discs. Ao, aorta.

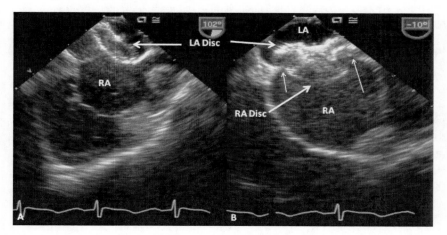

Figure 9. Selected two-dimensional video frames from a transesophageal echocardiographic study during the delivery of Amplatzer Septal Occluder in a different patient. Again, note thin arrows point to sandwiching of septal margins between LA and RA discs. Abbreviations are same as in figure 8.

Under echocardiographic guidance, the entire system is withdrawn such that the left atrial disk is flush against the left atrial side of the atrial septum occluding the ASD.

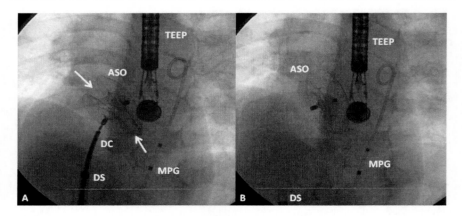

Figure 10. Selected cine frames from cineflurogram in a left axial oblique view $(30^0$ left anterior oblique and 30^0 cranial) demonstrating the position of the Amplatzer Septal Occluder (ASO) across the atrial septal defect prior to (A) and following (B) disconnecting the delivery cable (DC) from the ASO. Note the wide separation between discs (arrows). While this is not emphasized in the literature, we use this as another indicator for appropriate positioning of the device discs across the atrial septum in addition to visualization of septal rims sandwiched between left atrial and right atrial discs by transesophageal echocardiographic study as demonstrated in figures 8 and 9. DS, delivery sheath; MPG, marker pigtail catheter; TEEP, transesophageal echocardiography probe.

Then, while the device cable is held steady, the delivery sheath is withdrawn releasing the waist of the device within the atrial septal defect, followed by further withdrawal of the sheath deploying the right atrial disk in the right atrium (Figures 8B, 9B). The position of the device is verified by echocardiography and residual shunt looked for. Cinefluoroscopic appearance (Figure 10) of the device is also helpful in determining the adequacy of device placement. If the device position is satisfactory, the device cable is moved back and forth (so called Minnesota Wiggle). The position of the device is again verified by TEE (or ICE). If the device position is unsatisfactory, the device can be withdrawn into the sheath and redeployed. Once good device position is assured, the device cable is rotated counterclockwise and the device released. A repeat TEE/ICE to ensure good position of the device is undertaken (Figure 11). Complex ASDs including large defects, small septal rims, multiple defects and septal aneurysms pose additional problems and appropriate adjustments in the technique [34,35] may be necessary to ensure success of the device implantation in such defects.

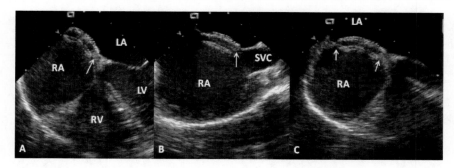

Figure 11. Selected two-dimensional video frames from a transesophageal echocardiographic study following the delivery of Amplatzer Septal Occluder demonstrating the position of both discs in four chamber (A), bi-caval (B) and long axis (C) views. Note that the rims of the defect (thin arrows) are sandwiched between left atrial (LA) and right atrial (RA) discs. LV, left ventricle; RV, right ventricle; SVC, superior vena cava.

Amplatzer Cribriform Device

Implantation of Amplatzer Cribriform Device is similar to that of Amplatzer Septal Occluder (Figures 12 and 13).

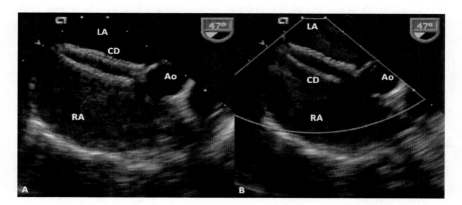

Figure 12. Selected two-dimensional video frame (A) and color frame (B) from a transesophageal echocardiographic study following the delivery of Amplatzer cribriform device (CD) demonstrating the position of both discs across the atrial septum (A) without any residual shunt (B) in a patient with fenestrated atrial septal defect shown in figures 5 and 6. Ao, aorta; LA, left atrium; RA, right atrium.

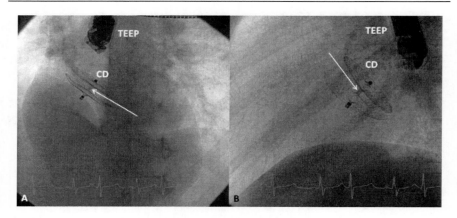

Figure 13. Selected cine frames from cineflurogram in a left axial oblique (30^0 left anterior oblique and 30^0 cranial) (A) and lateral (B) views demonstrating the position of the Amplatzer cribriform device (CD) across the fenestrated atrial septal defect in the patient shown in figures 5, 6 and 12. Note the thin waist (arrows in A and B) connecting the left and right atrial discs. Whereas the mechanism for atrial septal occlusion with Amplatzer Septal Occluder is by stenting the atrial septal defect with the waist of the device, the mechanism for occlusion of fenestrated atrial septal defect is by covering the defect with discs of the CD. TEEP, transesophageal echocardiography probe.

The delivery sheath should be positioned in the middle fenestration of the defect and the discs should cover the most peripheral fenestration to produce effective occlusion.

HELEX Device

The method of implantation is detailed elsewhere [36]. In brief, the delivery catheter (Green) is positioned in the left atrium over a guide wire and the wire withdrawn. Push-pinch-pull method is used to form the left atrial disk. Once the disk is formed, it is pulled back gently to engage the left side of the atrial septum, under fluoroscopic (Figure 14A) and TEE or ICE (Figure 15A) guidance. Then the delivery (Green) catheter is withdrawn over the control (Gray) catheter until the mandrel (Tan) engages the hub. Then the green catheter is fixed while the gray catheter is advanced to deliver the right atrial disk on the right side of the septum (Figure 14B and 15B), again using the "push-pinch-pull" technique.

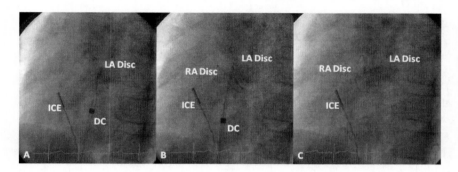

Figure 14. Selected cine frames from cineflurograms in a 60^0 left anterior oblique view demonstrating the position of the HELEX device following the delivery of the left atrial (LA) and right atrial (RA) discs and after disconnecting the delivery catheter (DC), respectively in A, B and C. Intra-cardiac echocardiography catheter (ICE) is seen with which ICE images shown in figure 15 are recorded.

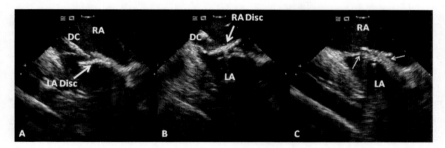

Figure 15. Selected two-dimensional video frames from an intra-cardiac echocardiographic study during HELEX device implantation showing delivery of the left atrial disc (LA Disc) into the left atrium (A) and right atrial disc (RA Disc) into the right atrium (B). Following disconnection of delivery catheter (DC) from the device (C) the rims of the defect (thin arrows) are sandwiched between LA and RA discs.

Once the device position is verified by echocardiography (TEE or ICE), the device is locked and then released (Figure 14 C and 15C).

IMMEDIATE AND FOLLOW-UP RESULTS

Amplatzer Septal Occluder

Immediate and mid-term follow-up results of Amplatzer Septal Occluder appear excellent with immediate complete closure rates varying from 62% to

96% which improved to 83% to 99% at six to 12 month follow-up [37]. A number of other studies have since been published and reveal similar results. We undertook closure of 150 ostium secundum defects with this device; there was a small residual shunt in two patients at the conclusion of the procedure. These shunt disappeared at one and six month follow-up visits respectively. No residual shunts observed during a follow-up of one to 60 months.

Device migration and erosion of aorta was observed during follow-up in 18 out of 15,900 (0.12% or 1 in 1,000) Amplatzer device implants in the US study population [38,39]. This complication was also similar (37 out of 35,000 - 0.11% or 1 in 1,000) in Amplatzer implants world-wide [38-40]. Review of data by the Review Board and AGA Medical (AGA 2006) suggested that the device erosion is related to over-sizing of the device and suggested that device size >1.5 times the TEE/ICE diameter of ASD should not be used.

Amplatzer Cribriform Device

There is limited published information on the results of this device (30,31,41). In one study [41], thirteen of sixteen patients had successful cribriform device closure. Complete closure was demonstrated in 77% of patients on the day following the procedure and 92% of patients at six and 12 months after the procedure. Figures 12 and 13 illustrate the cribriform device occlusion of fenestrated defect.

HELEX Device

Results of the multicenter trial [42] suggest successful implantation in 87% patients with low incidence (2.6%) of residual leaks at one year follow-up. Other reports suggest similar results. There was modest (8%) incidence of wire frame fractures. Helex device is generally considered to be a good device for occlusion of small to medium-sized ASDs. Figures 14 and 15 illustrate the HELEX device occlusion of a small atrial septal defect.

SURGICAL VS TRANSCATHETER CLOSURE

Though limited in number, the studies comparing surgical with device closure suggest similar effectiveness [43-46]. However, the device closure is less invasive, requiring no thoracotomy, cardio-pulmonary bypass and cardiotomy. The device closure also appears to have less number of complications (10% vs. 31%), require less hospital stay (1 day vs. 4.3 days), and is less expensive (US $ 11,000 vs. $ 21,000) [47]. The device closure techniques proved to be safe, cost-effective and favorably compare with surgical closure [43-48]. Transcatheter occlusion of ASDs using various devices is now an established practice in most centers providing state of the art care to patients with heart disease [35,49].

CONCLUSION

In this review clinical features and management of ostium secundum ASDs are discussed. Patients with ASDs, especially in childhood, are usually asymptomatic. Physical findings include hyperdynamic precordium, widely split and fixed second heart sound, ejection systolic murmur at the left upper sternal border and a mid-diastolic flow rumble at the left lower sternal border. Clinical diagnosis is not usually difficult and the diagnosis can be confirmed by non-invasive echocardiographic studies. Whereas surgical intervention was used in the past, transcatheter methods are currently used for closure of ostium secundum ASDs. While surgical closure is safe and effective, device closure carries less morbidity. Multiple devices have been investigated over the last few decades, but only Amplatzer (Septal Occluder and Cribriform) and HELEX devices received FDA approval as of this time. The Amplatzer Septal Occluder is useful in most ASDs while the HELEX device is useful in small and medium-sized defects. Amplatzer cribriform is useful in the occlusion of fenestrated defects. Amplatzer device appears to be best available option for most ostium secundum ASDs at the present time. Serious late complications may occur in 1 in 1,000 Amplatzer device implantations and these are likely to be avoided by keeping the device size < 1.5 times the size of ASD diameter on TEE/ICE. Careful attention to the details of the technique is mandatory to achieve a successful outcome.

REFERENCES

[1] Chopra, P. S.; Rao, PS. History of development of atrial septal occlusion devices, *Current Intervent Cardiol. Reports* 2000; 2:63-69.

[2] Rao, P. S. History of atrial septal occlusion devices. In: Catheter Based Devices for Treatment of Noncoronary Cardiovascular Disease in Adults and Children, Rao, P.S.; Kern, M.J. (Eds.): Lippincott, Williams and Wilkins, Philadelphia, PA, USA, 2003:1-9.

[3] King, T. D.; Mills, N. L. Nonoperative closure of atrial septal defects. *Surgery* 1974; 75:383-388.

[4] Mills, N.L.; King, T. D. Nonoperative closure of left-to-right shunts. *J. Thorac. Cardiovasc. Surg.* 1976; 72:371-378.

[5] King, T. D.; Thompson, S. L.; Steiner, C, et al. Secundum atrial septal defect: nonoperative closure during cardiac catheterization. *J. Am. Med. Assoc.* 1976; 235:2506-2509.

[6] Rashkind, W. J. Experimental transvenous closure of atrial and ventricular septal defects. *Circulation* 1975; 52:II-8.

[7] Rashkind, W. J.; Cuaso, C. E. Transcatheter closure of atrial septal defects in children. *Eur. J. Cardiol.* 1977; 8:119-120.

[8] Rashkind, W. J. Transcatheter treatment of congenital heart disease. *Circulation* 1983; 67:711-716.

[9] Rashkind, W. J.; Mullins, C. E.; Hellenbrand, W. E.; et alNon-surgical closure of patent ductus arteriosus: clinical applications of the Rashkind PDA occluder system. *Circulation* 1987; 75: 583-592.

[10] Lock, J. E.; Rome, J. J.; Davis, et al. Transcatheter closure of atrial septal defects: experimental studies. *Circulation* 1989; 79:1091-1099.

[11] Rome, J. J.; Keane, J. F.; Perry, S. B.; et al. Double-umbrella closure of atrial defects: initial clinical applications. *Circulation* 1990; 82: 751-758.

[12] Justo, R. N.; Nykanen, D. G.; Boutin, C.; et al Clinical impact of transcatheter closure of secundum atrial septal defects with the double umbrella device. *Am. J. Cardiol.* 1996; 77:889-892.

[13] Prieto, L. R.; Foreman, C. K.; Cheatham, J. P.; Latson, L. A. Intermediate-term outcome of transcatheter secundum atrial septal defect closure using the Bard Clamshell Septal Umbrella. *Am. J. Cardiol.* 1996; 78:1310-1312.

[14] Sideris, E. B.; Sideris, S. E.; Fowlkes, J. P.; et al. Transvenous atrial septal occlusion in piglets using a "buttoned" double-disc device. *Circulation* 1990; 81:312-318.

[15] Sideris, E. B.; Sideris, S. E.; Thanopoulos, B. D.; et al. Transvenous atrial septal defect occlusion by the "buttoned" device. *Am. J. Cardiol.* 1990; 66:1524-1526.

[16] Rao, P. S.; Wilson, A. D.; Levy, J. M.; et al. Role of "buttoned" double-disc device in the management of atrial septal defects. *Am. Heart J.* 1992; 123:191-200.

[17] Rao, P. S.; Sideris, E. B.; Hausdorf, G.; et al. International experience with secundum atrial septal defect occlusion by the buttoned device. *Am. Heart J.* 1994; 128:1022-1035.

[18] Rao, P. S.; Berger, F.; Rey, C.; et al. Transvenous occlusion of secundum atrial septal defects with 4th generation buttoned device: comparison with 1st, 2nd and 3rd generation devices. *J. Am. Coll Cardiol.* 2000; 36:583-592.

[19] Rao, P. S.; Sideris, E. B.; Haddad, J.; et al. Transcatheter occlusion of patent ductus arteriosus with adjustable buttoned device: initial clinical experience. *Circulation* 1993; 88:1119-1126.

[20] Sideris, E. B.; Leung, M.; Yoon, J. H.; et al. Occlusion of large atrial septal defects with a centering device: early clinical experience. *Am. Heart J.* 1996; 131:356-359.

[21] Rao, P. S.; Chander, J. S. and Sideris, E. B. Role of inverted buttoned device in transcatheter occlusion of atrial septal defects or patent foramen ovale with right-to-left shunting associated with previously operated complex congenital cardiac anomalies. *Am. J. Cardiol.* 1997; 80:914-921.

[22] Sideris, E. B.; Rey, C.; Schrader, R.; et al. Occlusion of large atrial septal defects by buttoned devices; comparison of centering and the fourth generation devices [abstract]. *Circulation* 1997; 96:(No. 8S) I-99.

[23] Rao, P. S.; Sideris, E. B. Centering-on-demand buttoned device: Its role in transcatheter occlusion of atrial septal defects. *J. Intervent Cardiol.* 2001; 14:81-89.

[24] Rao, P. S. Buttoned Device. In: Catheter based devices for the treatment of non-coronary cardiovascular disease in adults and children, P. S. Rao and M. J. Kern (Eds): Lippincott Williams and Wilkins, Philadelphia, PA, USA, 2003: 17-34.

[25] Ende, D. J.; Chopra, P. S.; Rao, P. S. Prevention of recurrence of paradoxical embolism: mid-term follow-up after transcatheter closure of atrial defects with buttoned device. *Am. J. Cardiol.* 1996; 78:233-236.

[26] Rao, P. S.; Palacios, I. F.; Bach, R. G.; et al. Platypnea- Orthodeoxia
      Syndrome: Management   by   Transcatheter   Buttoned   Device
      Implantation. *Cathet Cardiovasc Intervent* 2001; 54:77-82.

[27] Alapati, S.; Rao, P. S. Historical aspects of transcatheter occlusion of
      atrial septal defects. In: Rao, P. S. (ed): Atrial Septal Defects, InTech,
      Rijeka, Croatia, 2012:57-84.

[28] Rao, P. S. Historical aspects of therapeutic catheterization. In: Rao, P. S.
      (ed): Transcatheter Therapy in Pediatric Cardiology, Wiley-Liss, New
      York, NY, 1993:1-6.

[29] Sharafuddin, M. J. A.; Gu, X.; Titus, J. L.; et al. Transvenous closure of
      secundum atrial septal defects: preliminary results with a new self-
      expanding Nitinol prosthesis in a swine model. *Circulation* 1997;
      95:2162-2168.

[30] Hijazi, Z. M.; Cao, Q-L. Transcatheter closure of multi-fenestrated atrial
      septal defects using the new Amplatzer cribriform device. *Congenital
      Cardiology Today*, 2003; 1(1):1-4.

[31] Zanchetta, M.; Rigatelli, G.; Pedon, L.; et al. Catheter closure of
      perforated   secundum   atrial   septal   defect   under   intracardiac
      echocardiographic guidance using a single Amplatzer device: feasibility
      of a new method. *J. Invasive Cardiol.* 2005; 17: 262-265.

[32] Zahn, E.; Cheatham, J.; Latson, L.; Wilson, N. Results of in vivo testing
      of a new Nitinol ePTTEF septal occlusion device. *Cathet Cardiovasc.
      Intervent* 1999; 47:124.

[33] Carcagnì, A.; Presbitero, P. New echocardiographic diameter for
      Amplatzer sizing in adult patients with secundum atrial septal defect:
      preliminary results,. *Catheter Cardiovasc. Interv.* 2004; 62:409-414.

[34] Nagm, A. M.; Rao, P. S. Percutaneous occlusion of complex atrial septal
      defects. *J Invasive Cardiol* 2004: 16:123-125.

[35] Rao, P. S. Why, when and how should atrial septal defects be closed in
      adults. In: Rao, P. S. (ed): Atrial Septal Defects, InTech, Rijeka, Croatia,
      2012:121-138.

[36] Latson, LA.; Wilson, N.; Zahn, E. M. Helex septal occluder. In: Catheter
      Based Devices for Treatment of Noncoronary Cardiovascular Disease in
      Adults and Children, P.S. Rao, M.J. Kern. (Eds.): Lippincott, Williams
      and Wilkins, Philadelphia, PA, USA, 2003:71-78.

[37] Hamdan, M. A.; Cao, Q.; Hijazi, Z. M. Amplatzer septal occluder, In:
      Catheter Based Devices for Treatment of Noncoronary Cardiovascular
      Disease in Adults and Children, Rao, P.S.; Kern, M.J. (Eds.): Lippincott,
      Williams and Wilkins, Philadelphia, PA, USA, 2003:51-59.

[38] Amin, Z.; Hijazi, Z. M.; Bass, J. L.; et al. Erosion of Amplatzer septal occluder device after closure of secundum atrial septal defect: Review of registry of complications and recommendations to minimize future risk. *Cathet Cardiovascu Intervent* 2004; 63:491-502.

[39] AGA Medical Technical Note, January 2006:1-4.

[40] Crawford, G. B.; Brindis, R. G.; Krucoff, M. W.; et al. Percutaneous atrial Septal Occluder devices and cardiac erosion: A review of the literature. *Cathet Cardiovascu Intervent* 2012; 80:157-167

[41] Numan, M.; El Sisi, A.; Tofeig, M.; et al. (2008) Cribriform Amplatzer device closure of fenestrated atrial septal defects: feasibility and technical aspects. *Pediatr. Cardiol.* 2008; 29:530-535.

[42] Jones, T. K.; Latson, L. A.; Zahn, E.; et al. Multicenter Pivotal Study of the HELEX Septal Occluder Investigators. Results of the U.S. multicenter pivotal study of the HELEX septal occluder for percutaneous closure of secundum atrial septal defects, *J. Am. Coll Cardiol.* 2007; 49:2215-2221.

[43] Berger, F.; Vogel, M.; Alexi-Meskishvili, V.; Lange, P. E. Comparison of results and complications of surgical and Amplatzer device closure of atrial septal defects. *J. Thorac. Cardiovasc. Surg.* 1999; 118:674-678.

[44] Du, Z. D.; Hijazi, Z. M.; Kleinman, C.S.; et al. Comparison between transcatheter and surgical closure of secundum atrial septal defect in children and adults: results of multicenter nonrandomized trial. *J. Am. Coll Cardiol.* 2002; 39:1836-1844.

[45] Durongpisitkul, K.; Soongswang, J.; Laohaprasitiporn, D.; et al. Comparison of atrial septal defect closure using Amplatzer septal occluder with surgery. *Pediatr. Cardiol.* 2002; 23:36-40.

[46] Bialkowski, J.; Karwot, B.; Szkutnik, M.; et al. Closure of atrial septal defects in children: surgery versus Amplatzer device implantation. *Tex Heart Inst. J.* 2004; 31:220-223.

[47] Kim, J. J.; Hijazi, Z. M. Clinical outcomes and costs of Amplatzer transcatheter closure as compared with surgical closure of ostium secundum atrial septal defects. *Med. Science Monitor* 2002; 8:CR787-791.

[48] Bettencourt, N.; Salome, N.; Carneiro, F.; et al. Atrial septal closure in adults: surgery versus Amplatzer—comparison of results. *Rev. Port Cardiol.* 2003; 22:1203-1211.

[49] Rao, P. S. Catheter Closure of Atrial Septal Defects (Editorial). *J. Invasive Cardiol.* 2003; 15:398-400.

In: Atrial and Ventricular Septal Defects
Editor: Steven A. Larkin

ISBN: 978-1-62618-326-1
© 2013 Nova Science Publishers, Inc.

Chapter 4

ATRIAL AND VENTRICULAR SEPTAL DEFECTS: ETIOLOGY AND PERCUTANEOUS CLOSURE

José F. Díaz Fernández, Carlos Sánchez-González Antonio Gómez-Menchero, Jessica Roa Garrido, Rosa Cardenal Piris and Ana José Manovel Sánchez*

Cardiology and Vascular Surgery Unit, Juan Ramon
Jimenez Hospital, Huelva, Spain

ABSTRACT

Atrial and ventricular septal defects (AVSD) are the most frequent congenital heart defects, affecting a 0.5% of new-borns. Their etiology includes a variety of causes, from genetic or genomic variation to the exposure to environment factors.

Among AVSD there are two well differentiated scenarios: 1) syndromic AVSD (Down syndrome or Holt-Oram syndrome) where genetic disturbances are the main reason for the development of the condition, and 2) non syndromic AVSD where the interaction between genetic predisposition and environment factors affects critically biological systems during heart development.

* Corresponding author: Carlos Sánchez-González. E-mail: coxibum@hotmail.com.

Genetic predisposition is not always fully characterized although some specific genetic features like carrying MDR1 3435CT/TT genotype or NNMT A allele have been proven an additional risk for developing non syndromic AVSD. This risk can be higher when some types of environment factors get combined, including cigarette smoking, benzodyacepines, alcohol and serotonin reuptake inhibitors consumption and the exposure to air pollution. All of these are present often in daily life, constituting a reason for great concern.

The association between environment factors and the development of AVSD has been repeteadly shown in different studies; for instance, cigarette smoking during pregnancy causes a three-fold increase in the risk of AVSD. The majority of this studies are, however, retrospective epidemiological studies, what carries a great limitation for the interpretation of results. Therefore, prospective cohort studies would be paramount to get more definite conclusions about the influence of environment factors in the development of AVSD.

The extraordinary development of medical devices has made possible the percutaneous (non surgical) treatment of atrial and ventricular septal defects in many cases.

In the case of atrial septal defects (ASD), percutaneous closure is mainly indicated for ostium secundum defects although other types of ASD can also be treated percutaneously. In order to establish correctly the indication of closure both right cardiac catheterization and echocardiography are critical, not only for patient selection but for guidance and assistance during the closure procedure.

Several ASD ocluders are clinically available (Amplatzer[tm], Gore Helex[tm], STARFlex[tm], Premere[tm]...) all of them consisting of two discs separated by a waist. In general, the vast majority of ASD can be treated percutaneously with reasonably small sheats (12 french or less). Success rates are very high (98-99% after three months of follow up) and complications (device embolization, pericardial effusion or trombosis) are usually below 1%.

Regarding ventricular septal defects (VSD) percutaneous treatment is not so widely used. Post-myocardial infarction VSD with a very high surgical risk and selected cases of perimembranous VSD are the ones treated more commonly. With a correct case selection, percutaneous closure of VSD is a safe and feasible procedure, although small residual left to right shunts are observed in a relatively high percentage of patients.

INTRODUCTION

Atrial and ventricular septal defects (AVSD) are common cardiovascular malformations reported in around 0,5% of newborns. In the current era, thanks to the success of paediatric cardiac care as well as the improvement in case ascertainment and reporting, there is an increase in the number of adult patients with AVSD. That implies a rise in both the prevalence and the burden of AVSD that may lead to the development of new strategies to control this increasing sanitary problem.

There are two well differentiated scenarios where AVSD can occur: 1) syndromic AVSD, where cardiac malformations appear directly as a result of a genetic abnormality or are strongly associated with and underlying genetic disorder (Down syndrome, Holt-Oram syndrome), and 2) non syndromic AVSD where the condition is directly related to the effect of an environmental toxin (e.g., alcohol or tobacco) or, which is most common, results from an interaction between multifactorial genetic and environmental influences.

In order to reduce the burden of these conditions it is important to know their etiologic factors, particularly those modifiable related to environmental situations as avoiding the exposure to them may lead to a decrease in the incidence of AVSD.

Therefore, this review summarizes environmental factors for AVSD and the corresponding strategies to reduce the risk of developing cardiac malformations. Apart from that, genetic factors and some examples of interaction between environment and genetic predisposition are presented as well as the main advances in non surgical/percutaneous treatment of AVSD which are of great interest as they provide important advantages for these patients in comparison with traditional surgical treatment.

GENETIC AND MOLECULAR DETERMINANTS

Although most cardiovascular malformations are not inherited in a simple manner, there are some of them strongly associated with an underlying genetic disorder where the genes responsible have been clearly identified.

Those genes have also been cloned, and the knowledge of their products has provided insights into the disease processes as well as the pathways regulating cardiac development. These most representative AVSD syndrome are the following:

Down Syndrome

This entity is particularly associated with one type of AVSD, the commonly referred to as endocardial cushion or atrioventricular canal defects. This is characterized by varying degrees of incomplete development of those structures derived from endocardial cushion (inferior portion of the atrial septum, the inflow portion of the ventricular septum, and atrioventricular valves) and can be found around 40% of patients with the syndrome. The hypothesized mechanism responsible for this alteration seems to consist of duplications of small region of chromosome 21 that lead to an overdose of some specific genes responsible for avoiding the normal development of structures derived from endocardial cushion [1, 2]. As it is discussed later, some environmental factors like maternal tobacco consumption may play a role in modulating the likelihood of developing the cardiac defect among patients with Down Syndrome.

Holt-Oram Syndrome

It is one of the best known syndrome AVSD. Abnormalities of the upper limbs together with single or several AVSD are the main findings as well as cardiac conduction defects which are also frequently present. The gen involved is named TBX5 for which a large number of mutations have been identified, however only some of them have been found to cause skeletal and cardiac malformations. The cell-specific effects of TBX5 mutations are largely unknown but it seems that it produces an inhibition in cardiomyocite proliferation and therefore in the process of cardiogenesis including trabecullation and cardiac septation [3].

Ellis-Van Creveld Syndrome

Like Holt-Oram syndrome, this is another example of the association of cardiac septal defects with skeletal deformity. Atrial septal defects is typically associated with other anomalies like shortening of extremities, polydactyly or upper lip deformity. Positional cloning studies have identified the gene responsible for the syndrome in the chromosome 4p16.1. However, the specific molecular roles and cellular functions modulating atrial septation in Ellis-van Creveld Syndrome remain to be elucidated [4].

Another important gene in the process of septation during cardiac morphogenesis is NKX2. Mutations in this gene has been found in some types of familial AVSD, frequently associated with progressive atrioventricular block as the gene is also important for the maintenance of atrioventricular node function throughout life [5].

There are other genetic profiles, not always fully characterized, that implies some type of genetic predisposition like carrying MDR1 3435CT/TT genotype or NNMT A allele which have been demonstrated to imply an additional risk of developing non syndrome AVSD.

ENVIRONMENTAL FACTORS

The important socioeconomic transformation occurred during the last decades in developing countries implies deep changes in both the environment and the style of life. Health consequences derived from these changes are usually difficult to predict and detect as they usually consist of uncommon disorders or diseases with a long latency period. However, as they have a ubiquitous distribution, small increases in risk may therefore carry a large public health implication.

In the case of cardiac septal defects there are some well established traditional environmental factors like maternal rubella or the ingestion of some drugs early in gestation such as thalidomide or isotretinoin. However, with the current status of society in the western countries, there are others environmental factors with a probably much higher impact in terms of public health costs. Some of these important factors are the following: air pollution, maternal smoking, alcohol consumption and maternal diabetes.

Air Pollution

There is a growing body of epidemiologic evidence thorough the last decade which suggest associations between air pollution and cardiac septal defects. In the case-control study by Ritz et al., they found that carbon monoxide exposure during pregnancy increased the frequency of ventricular septal defects in a dose-response fashion [6]. In the same manner, Gilboa et al. reported positive associations between small particulate matter and sulphur dioxide during pregnancy with the development of isolated atrial septal defect and ventricular septal defect respectively [7]. Nevertheless, uncertainties still remain concerning the effects of specific pollutants as there are some studies like the reported by Strickland et al. where no association was found between the level of more than 60 air pollutions and the risk of cardiovascular malformations [8]. Or the case-control study by Lupo et al., specifically designed to confirm the relation between cardiac septal defects and maternal exposure to polycyclic aromatic hydrocarbons, that could not reach its primary target [9].

There are many factors that could explain the above mentioned inconsistencies like the high variability of levels and quality of air pollutants among different regions, the differences in the definition of exposure including the window of exposure, out-door vs indoor exposure, etc. and the difficulties to adjust for potential confounders given the nature of the study design in the majority of cases, usually retrospective case-control studies.

Several mechanisms have been hypothesized for teratogenicity of air pollutants including oxidative stress, placental inflammation, and changes in coagulation; these may affect early fetal growth influencing the migration and differentiation of neural crest cells [10].

The strategies to control this sanitary problem should include further studies to define more accurately the role of the different air pollutants in the development of AVSD, identify those with the highest impact in public health and design measures to avoid the exposition of those factors to the most vulnerable population.

Maternal Smoking

Maternal active consumption of tobacco as well as passive tobacco exposure, has been related to an increased risk of septal defects in newborns, specially atrial septal defects in which the estimated relative risk increases with the number of cigarettes smoked [11, 12, 13]. No association has been found so far between maternal smoking and endocardial cushion defects or ventricular septal defects.

Possible mechanisms of teratogenicity of smoking remain speculative, but most scientists report that toxic compounds in smoke have adverse effects on organogenesis including fetal hypoxia caused by carbon monoxide, impaired uteroplacental circulation with resultant reduced supply of essential nutrients for embryonic tissues and DNA damage from polycyclic aromatic hydrocarbons.

The evidence of a relation between tobacco exposure and cardiac septal defects is of great importance for public health as smoking is one of the most preventable risk factor. In fact, with the growing evidence about the effect of smoking during pregnancy and the benefits of smoking cessation, specially during first trimester, women are now more likely to stop their smoking behaviours. However, they might be also more reluctant to admit to smoking during pregnancy, a circumstance that leads to a misclassification which effects are unpredictable [14].

Alcohol Consumption

Alcohol is the teratogenic most frequently and widely used worldwide. According to recent epidemiological studies, more than 10% of pregnant women drink alcohol, a feature with great public health implications as alcohol exposure during pregnancy has been associated with congenital heart disease, even when it happens during few days, as reported by Webster et al. [15].

The role of alcohol in humans as an independent cause of cardiac malformations is often difficult to establish as it commonly coexist with other situations strongly associated with the development of cardiac congenital abnormalities like low cultural level or teenage pregnancy. In any case, it seems clear that alcohol has a teratogenitiy effect by several mechanisms including among others the apoptosis and subsequent losses of cardiac neural crest populations [16] and the induction of embryonic oxidative stress. All these disturbances lead to the called fetal alcohol syndrome which consist of a large number of serius anomalies including cardiac septal defects and more specifically ventricular septal defect.

Given de addictive nature of alcohol consumption, health public strategies based on information and motivation for alcohol-consuming mothers are likely to be unsuccessful. An alternative approach that should be seriously considered in this population is the administration of the antioxidants vitamin C and E, as it has been found in previous studies to reduce significantly fetal alcohol damage [17].

Maternal Diabetes

Maternal diabetes has been independently linked to a higher risk of bearing infants with congenital cardiac malformations, with a worse clinical profile and a poorer prognosis including a higher frequency of extracardiac anomalies, low birth weight and mortality. The typical cardiac anomaly linked to maternal diabetes is hypertrophic cardiomyopathy, a pathology that has been related to hiperinsulinism wheter or not there is reasonable metabolic control. But apart from that condition, which usually regresses within months after birth, maternal diabetes has been also related to other congenital heart defects including cardiac septal defects and more importantly ventricular septal defects.

Unlike hypertrophic cardiomyopathy, the likelihood of developing cardiac septal defects seems to be influenced by metabolic control. High maternal haemoglobin A1c values during early pregnancy are associated with increased risk of malformations and hyperglycemia has a direct influence on the proliferation and migration of neural crest cells which are critical in the development of the heart.

These features are of great and urgent clinical significance as the effectiveness of early preconceptional care in the prevention of congenital anomalies has been demonstrated repeatedly [18].

INTERACTION OF ENVIRONMENTAL AND GENETIC FACTORS

Apart from direct influence of environmental factors, the majority of studies suggest that influences of the environment usually interact with genetic predisposition leading to a modification in the likelihood of having cardiac malformations. One classical example is Down syndrome where environmental factors can interact with trisomic genome to modulate the risk of developing AVSD and other associated anomalies, for instance maternal tobacco consumption as it was seen in the study by Torfs et al., they found a higher frequency of septal cardiac defects among Down syndrome patients when maternal tobacco consumption coexisted [19]. Apart from Down syndrome, there are others genetic susceptibilities in some individuals which make them more vulnerable to the adverse effects of tobacco like genetic polymorphisms in the nitric oxide synthasa gene which leads to a deficiency in the enzyme oxide xynthasa. That is a system with important biological functions like vasodilation, angiogenesis and also heart development; therefore its deficiency implies a high vulnerability for the development of cardiac malformations including AVSD. This vulnerability is also specially high when maternal smoking coexist [20].

In the opposite sense, environmental factors can also interact with genetic or genomic variation decreasing the likelihood of cardiovascular malformations. One typical example is using folic acid supplements during gestation, Obermann et al. found that mothers carrying the MDR1 3435T allele, a genomic variation that implies a nearly 3-fold increased risk for cardiac septal defects, diminished significantly its risk, nearly up to its neutralization, when consuming folic acid supplements [21, 22]

All these features are essential for public health, which to build clinical and public health primary prevention strategies. It is important to emphasize on the need to instruct the public about the importance of pre-marital counselling and the deleterious effects of various teratogens in the environment. Physicians who treat pregnant women should be aware of the effects of known teratogens, avoid those agents and provide interventions like folic acid administration or vitamin supplements of proven efficacy in the prevention of cardiovascular and other malformations.

Aditionally, detection of genetic abnormalities during fetal life from amniotic fluid or chorionic villus biopsy is becoming and increasing reality.

NON-SURGICAL INTERVENTIONS

The extraordinary development of Interventional Cardiology has made possible the percutaneous treatment of some AVSD. We will focus on two specific entities, the *secundum* atrial septal defect (SASD) and the *muscular* ventricular septal defect, that are the only two ones in which a percutaneous closure can be indicated.

Atrial Septal Defect Closure

An ASD, the most frequent congenital heart disease in adults, is a persistent communication between the atria. There are several different types of ASD: the secundum ASD in the región of the fossa ovalis (75% of cases), the primum ASD (15% to 20%) positioned inferiorly near the crux of the heart, the sinus venosus ASD (5% to 10%) located superiorly near the superior vena caval entry or inferiorly near the inferior vena caval entry, and the uncommon coronary sinus septal defect (less than 1%), which causes shunting through the ostium of the coronary sinus [22]. Only SASD is the type of ASD indicated for percutaneous closure (non-surgical), what is being done since 1990 [23].

Transesophageal echocardiography (TEE) is used to confirm the presence of an SASD and to characterize it, visualizing the entire atrial septum and assessing the number of orifices (single or fenestrated), the location and dimensions (measured in two planes) and morphology of the SASD, its rims and anatomical relationships, and associated lesions. Conventionally, the rims of a SASD are labeled as aortic (superoanterior), atrioventricular (AV) valve (mitral or inferoanterior), superior venacaval (SVC or superoposterior), inferior venacaval (IVC or inferoposterior), and posterior (from the posterior free wall of the atria). By conventional definition, a margin >5 mm is considered to be adequate for percutaneous closure. (Figure 1).

Several devices have been used, including the CardioSEAL/STARFlex devices, the Sideris buttoned device, the HELEX device and the Amplatzer Septal Occluder (ASO, AGA Medical). The ASO has become the most widely used because of its high closure rates, safety of use, ease of deployment and eventual retrieval, and ability to close large defects. It consists a nitinol structure of two discs that convey in a central waist (figure 2).

In a recent meta-analysis [24] of more tan 3000 patients, percutaneous and surgical closure of ASD were compared. A very low rate of complications was observed with both modalities, although percutaneous closure showed a significantly lower number of complications (6.6 vs 31%, p<0.05), being the embolisation or malposition of the device the most common one in the precutaneous group.

Long-term prognosis after percutaneous closure is usually excellent [25] and most patients remain free of symptoms and without significant right ventricule dilation, arrythmias or pulmonary hypertension.

Ventricular Septal Defect Closure

Ventricular septal defect (VSD) is one of the commonest congenital malformations of the heart, accounting for up to 40% of all cardiac anomalies [26]. Broadly speaking, defects can be classified according to their location, either within the muscular septum (muscular defects) or at its margins. Ventricular septal defects at the margins of the muscular septum can be related to hinge-points of the leaflets of the atrioventricular valves (perimembranous), those of the arterial valves (juxta-arterial or subarterial), or both.

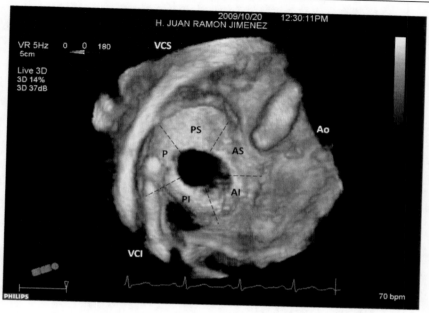

Figure 1. D TEE picture of a centrally located ostium secundum atrial septal defect and its anatomical relationships as seen from the right atrium. The rims (AS: antero-superior; PS: postero-superior; P: posterior; PI: postero-inferior; AI: antero-inferior) and their position related to the superior (VCS) and inferior vena cava (VCI), and aorta (Ao) are shown.

Transcatheter closure can be considered in patients with increased risk factors for surgery, multiple previous cardiac surgical interventions, or VSDs that are poorly accessible for surgical closure. In muscular VSDs that are located centrally in the interventricular septum, it can be considered as an alternative to surgical closure. In perimembranous VSD it has been shown to be feasible. The Amplatzer VSD closure device is the most widely used (figure 3). The results of percutaneous closure are encouraging; in 2004, the United States registry of the Amplatzer Muscular VSD occluder reported 83 procedures in 75 patients with a median age of 1.4 years, who underwent percutaneous (70 of 75) and/or perventricular (6 of 75) closure of hemodynamically significant congenital single or multiple muscular VSDs [27]. The device was implanted successfully in 72 of the 83 (86.7%) procedures. Major procedure- or device-related complications occurred in 10.7% of the patients. Closure rates were excellent and increased from 47.2% 24 hours post-procedure to 92.3% at 12 months' follow-up.

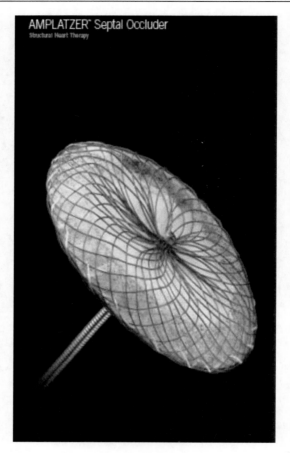

Figure 2. Amplatzer ASD closure device, AGA Medical.

Closure rates were excellent and increased from 47.2% 24 hours post-procedure to 92.3% at 12 months' follow-up.

In 2005, Thanopoulos reported intermediate-term outcome in 30 children with single muscular VSD. Successful closure of the defect was achieved in 28 of the 30 patients (93%).

Major complication was noted in only one patient (4.2 kg) who developed a complete heart block [28].

In conclusion, transcatheter closure of muscular VSDs using the Amplatzer muscular VSD occluders is effective and safe. It has no scar, less pain, shorter hospital stay, and less cost compared with the traditional open heart surgery.

Muscular

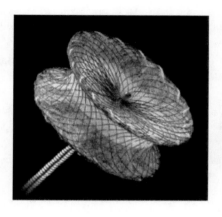

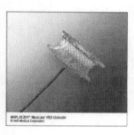

Muscular Post Infarto

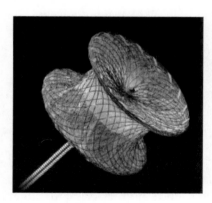

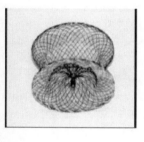

Figure 3. Amplatzer muscular VSD closure device, AGA Medical.

We would like to finish by stating that the majority of information presented here comes from retrospective epidemiological studies, generally case-control studies, what carries a great limitation for the interpretation of results including added difficulties to control confounding factors. Therefore, prospective cohort studies would be paramount to get more definite conclusions about the influence of environment factors in the development of AVSD.

REFERENCES

[1]   Korenberg, J. R., Chen, X. N., Schipper, R., et al. 1994. Down syndrome phenotypes: the consequences of chromosomal imbalance. *Proc. Natl. Acad. Sci. US* 91:4997-5001.

[2]   Benson, D. W., Basson, C. T., MacRae, C. A. 1996. New understandings in the genetics of congenital heart disease. *Curr. Opin. Pediatr.* 8:505-511.

[3]   Kim, M. S., Hatcher, C. J., Wong, B., et al. 2000. Tbx5 transcription factor: a cellular arrest signal Turing vertebrate cardiogenesis. *Circulation* 102:100-110.

[4]   Ruiz-Pérez, V. L., Ide, S., Strom, T. M., et al. 2000. Mutations in a new gene in Ellis-van Creveld syndrome and Weyers acrodenal dysostosis. *Nat. Genet.* 24:283-286.

[5]   Benson, D. W., Silberbach, G. M., Kavanaugh-McHugh, A., et al. 1999. Mutations in the cardiac transcription factor NKX2.5 affect diverse cardiac developmental pathways. *J. Clin. Invest.* 104:1567-1573.

[6]   Ritz, B., Yu, F., Fruin, S., Chapa, G., et al. Ambient air pollution and risk of birth defects in Southern California. *Am. J. Epidemiol.* 2002 Jan. 1;155(1):17-25.

[7]   Gilboa, S. M., Mendolal, P., Olshan, A. F., et al. Relation between ambient air quality and selected birth defects, seven conty study, Texas, 1997-2000. *Am. J. Epidemiol.* 2005 Aug.;162(3):238-52.

[8]   Strickland, M. J., Klein, M., Correa, A., et al. Ambient air pollution and cardiovascular malformations in Atlanta, Georgia, 1986-2003. *Am. J. Epidemiol.* 2009 Apr. 15;169(8):1004-14. doi: 10.1093/aje/kwp011. Epub. 2009 Mar. 3.

[9]   Lupo, P. J., Symanski, E., Langlois, P. H. Maternal occupational exposure to polycyclic aromatic hydrocarbons and congenital heart defects among offspring in the national birth defects prevention study. *Birth Defects Res. A Clin. Mol. Teratol.* 2012 Nov.;94(11):875-81.

[10] Kannan, S., Misra, D. P., Dvonch, J. T., Krishnakumar, A. Exposures to airborne particulate matter and adverse perinatal outcomes: a biologically plausible mechanistic framework for exploring potential effect modification by nutrition. *Environ. Health Perspect.* 2006;114: 1636–1642.

[11] Renata Kučienė, Virginija Dulskienė. Parental cigarette smoking and the risk of congenital heart septal defects Medicina (Kaunas) 2010; 46(9): 635-41.

[12] Kallen, K. Maternal smoking and congenital heart defects. *Eur. J. Epidemiol.* 1999;15:731-7.

[13] Malik, S., Cleves, M. A., Honein, M. A Maternal smoking and congenital heart defects. *Pediatrics.* 2008 Apr.;121(4):e810-6.

[14] Colman, G. J., Joyce, T. Trends in smoking before, during, and after pregnancy in ten states. *Am. J. Prev. Med.* 2003;24(1):29–35.

[15] Webster, W., Ann Germain, M. A., Lipson, A., et al. Alcohol and congenital heart defects: an experimental study in mice. *Cardiovasc. Res.* (1984) 18(6).

[16] Cavieres, M. F. and Smith, S. M. (2000), Genetic and Developmental Modulation of Cardiac Deficits in Prenatal Alcohol Exposure. *Alcoholism: Clinical and Experimental Research*, 24: 102–109

[17] Cohen-Kerem, R., Koren, G. Antioxidants and fetal protection against ethanol teratogenicity. I. Review of the experimental data and implications to humans. *Neurotoxicol. Teratol.* 2003 Jan-Feb.;25(1):1-9.

[18] Loffredo, C. A., Hirata, J., Wilson, P. D., et al. Atrioventricular septal defects: possible etiologic differences between complete and partial defects. *Teratology* 2001 Feb.; 63(2):87-93.

[19] Torfs, C. P., Christianson, R. E. Maternal risk factors and major associated defects in infants with Down Syndrome. *Epidemiology.* 1999 May;10(3):264-70.

[20] Liu, Y., Feng, Q. NOing the heart: role of nitric oxide synthase-3 in heart development. *Differentiation.* 2012 Jl;84(1):54-61.

[21] Obermann-Borst, S. A., Isaacs, A., Younes, Z., et al. General maternal medication use, folic acid, the MDR1 c3435T polymorphism, and the risk of a child with a congenital heart defect. *Am. J. Obstet. Gynecol.* 2011 Mar.;204(3).

[22] Fuster, V., Brandenburg, R. O., McGoon, D. C., Giuliani, E. R. Clinical approach and management of congenital heart disease in the adolescent and adult. *Cardiovasc. Clin.* 1980;10:161–97.

[23] Rao, P. S., Wilson, A. D., Levy, J. M., Gupta, V. K., Chopra, P. S. Role of "buttoned" double-disc device in the management of atrial septal defects. *Am. Heart J.* 1992; 123(1):191-200.

[24] Butera, G., Biondi-Zoccai, G., Sangiorgi, G., et al. Percutaneous versus surgical closure of secundum atrial septal defects: a systematic review and meta-analysis of currently available clinical evidence. *Eurointervention* 2011; 7: 377-85.

[25] Kutty, S., Hazeem, A., Brown, K., et al. Long-Term (5- to 20-Year) Outcomes After Transcatheter or Surgical Treatment of

Hemodynamically Significant Isolated Secundum Atrial Septal Defect. *Am. J. Cardiol.* 2012; 109: 1348 –1352.

[26] Hoffman, J. I. Incidence of congenital heart disease: I—postnatal incidence. *Pediatr. Cardiol.* 1995; 16: 103–13.

[27] Holzer, R., Balzer, D., Cao, Q. L.,et al. Device closure of muscular ventricular septal defects using the Amplatzer muscular ventricular septal defect occluder: immediate and mid-term results of a US registry. *J. Am. Coll. Cardiol.* 2004;43: 1257e63.

[28] Thanopoulos, B. D. Catheter closure of congenital muscular ventricular septal defects. *Pediatr. Cardiol.* 2005; 26: 220e3.

INDEX

C

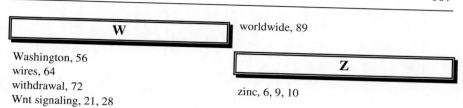

W

Washington, 56
wires, 64
withdrawal, 72
Wnt signaling, 21, 28

worldwide, 89

Z

zinc, 6, 9, 10